PROGRESS IN CLINICAL AND BIOLOGICAL RESEARCH

Vol 1: **Erythrocyte Structure and Function,** George J. Brewer, *Editor*

Vol 2: **Preventability of Perinatal Injury,** Karlis Adamsons and Howard A. Fox, *Editors*

Vol 3: **Infections of the Fetus and the Newborn Infant,** Saul Krugman and Anne A. Gershon, *Editors*

Vol 4: **Conflicts in Childhood Cancer,** Lucius F. Sinks and John O. Godden, *Editors*

Vol 5: **Trace Components of Plasma: Isolation and Clinical Significance,** G.A. Jamieson and T.J. Greenwalt, *Editors*

Vol 6: **Prostatic Disease,** H. Marberger, H. Haschek, H.K.A. Schirmer, J.A.C. Colston, and E. Witkin, *Editors*

Vol 7: **Blood Pressure, Edema and Proteinuria in Pregnancy,** Emanuel A. Friedman, *Editor*

Vol 8: **Cell Surface Receptors,** Garth L. Nicolson, Michael A. Raftery, Martin Rodbell, and C. Fred Fox, *Editors*

Vol 9: **Membranes and Neoplasia: New Approaches and Strategies,** Vincent T. Marchesi, *Editor*

Vol 10: **Diabetes and Other Endocrine Disorders During Pregnancy and in the Newborn,** Maria I. New and Robert H. Fiser, *Editors*

Vol 11: **Clinical Uses of Frozen-Thawed Red Blood Cells,** John A. Griep, *Editor*

Vol 12: **Breast Cancer,** Albert C.W. Montague, Geary L. Stonesifer, Jr., and Edward F. Lewison, *Editors*

Vol 13: **The Granulocyte: Function and Clinical Utilization,** Tibor J. Greenwalt and G.A. Jamieson, *Editors*

Vol 14: **Zinc Metabolism: Current Aspects in Health and Disease,** George J. Brewer and Ananda S. Prasad, *Editors*

Vol 15: **Cellular Neurobiology,** Zach Hall, Regis Kelly, and C. Fred Fox, *Editors*

Vol 16: **HLA and Malignancy,** Gerald P. Murphy, *Editor*

Vol 17: **Cell Shape and Surface Architecture,** Jean Paul Revel, Ulf Henning, and C. Fred Fox, *Editors*

Vol 18: **Tay-Sachs Disease: Screening and Prevention,** Michael M. Kaback, *Editor*

Vol 19: **Blood Substitutes and Plasma Expanders,** G.A. Jamieson and T.J. Greenwalt, *Editors*

Vol 20: **Erythrocyte Membranes: Recent Clinical and Experimental Advances,** Walter C. Kruckeberg, John W. Eaton, and George J. Brewer, *Editors*

Vol 21: **The Red Cell,** George J. Brewer, *Editor*

Vol 22: **Molecular Aspects of Membrane Transport,** Dale Oxender and C. Fred Fox, *Editors*

Vol 23: **Cell Surface Carbohydrates and Biological Recognition,** Vincent T. Marchesi, Victor Ginsburg, Phillips W. Robbins, and C. Fred Fox, *Editors*

Vol 24: **Twin Research,** Proceedings of 2nd International Congress on Twin Studies
Walter E. Nance, *Editor*
Published in 3 Volumes:
Part A: Psychology and Methodology
Part B: Biology and Epidemiology
Part C: Clinical Studies

Vol 25: **Recent Advances in Clinical Oncology,** Tapan A. Hazra and Michael C. Beachley, *Editors*

Vol 26: **Origin and Natural History of Cell Lines,** Claudio Barigozzi, *Editor*

Vol 27: **Membrane Mechanism of Drugs of Abuse,** Charles W. Sharp and Leo G. Abood, *Editors*

Vol 28: **The Blood Platelet in Transfusion Therapy,** G.A. Jamieson and Tibor J. Greenwalt, *Editors*

Vol 29: **Biomedical Applications of the Horseshoe Crab (Limulidae),** Elias Cohen, *Editor-in-Chief*

Vol 30: **Normal and Abnormal Red Cell Membranes,** Samuel E. Lux, Vincent T. Marchesi, and C. Fred Fox, *Editors*

Vol 31: **Transmembrane Signaling,** Mark Bitensky, R. John Collier, Donald F. Steiner, and C. Fred Fox, *Editors*

Vol 32: **Genetic Analysis of Common Diseases: Applications to Predictive Factors in Coronary Disease,** Charles F. Sing and Mark Skolnick, *Editors*

Vol 33: **Prostate Cancer and Hormone Receptors,** Gerald P. Murphy and Avery A. Sandberg, *Editors*

Vol 34: **The Management of Genetic Disorders,** Constantine J. Papadatos and Christos S. Bartsocas, *Editors*

Vol 35: **Antibiotics and Hospitals,** Carlo Grassi and Giuseppe Ostino, *Editors*

Vol 36: **Drug and Chemical Risks to the Fetus and Newborn,** Richard H. Schwarz and Sumner J. Yaffe, *Editors*

DRUG AND CHEMICAL RISKS TO THE FETUS AND NEWBORN

DRUG AND CHEMICAL RISKS TO THE FETUS AND NEWBORN

Proceedings of a Symposium Held in New York City, May 1979
Presented by the State University of New York, Downstate Medical Center
Sponsored by the National Foundation—March of Dimes

Editors

RICHARD H. SCHWARZ, MD
Professor and Chairman, Department of Obstetrics/Gynecology
State University of New York
Downstate Medical Center
Brooklyn, New York

and

SUMNER J. YAFFE, MD
University of Pennsylvania School of Medicine
Director, Division of Clinical Pharmacology
Children's Hospital
Philadelphia, Pennsylvania

ALAN R. LISS, INC., NEW YORK

Address all Inquiries to the Publisher
Alan R. Liss, Inc., 150 Fifth Avenue, New York, NY 10011

Printed in the United States of America

Library of Congress Cataloging in Publication Data

Main entry under title:

Drug and chemical risks to the fetus and newborn.

(Progress in clinical and biological research; v. 36)
Includes index.
1. Fetus, Effect of drugs on the – Congresses. 2. Teratogenic agents – Congresses. 3. Infants (Newborn) – Drug effects – Congresses. 4. Milk, Human – Contamination – Congresses. I. Schwarz, Richard H. II. Yaffe, Sumner J., 1923 - III. Series.
RG627.6.D79D78 618.3′2 79-26191
ISBN 0-8451-0036-X

Contents

Contributors

Cheston M. Berlin, Jr., Department of Pediatrics and Department of Pharmacology, Pennsylvania State University College of Medicine, Hershey, PA 17033 **(115)**

Alfred M. Bongiovanni, Department of Endocrinology, Catholic University of Puerto Rico, School of Medicine, Ponce Station 6, Puerto Rico 00731 **(139)**

Sanford N. Cohen, Department of Pediatrics, Wayne State University School of Medicine and Children's Hospital of Michigan, Detroit, MI 48201 **(129)**

Anke A. Ehrhardt, Department of Psychiatry, College of Physicians and Surgeons of Columbia University and New York State Psychiatric Institute, New York, NY 10032 **(93)**

Marion J. Finkel, Bureau of Drugs, Food and Drug Administration, Rockville, MD 20857 **(67)**

Martha M. Freeman, Bureau of Drugs, Food and Drug Administration, Rockville, MD 20857 **(67)**

Allen S. Goldman, Division of Teratology, The Children's Hospital of Philadelphia, Philadelphia, PA 19104 **(9)**

Donald E. Hutchings, Department of Behavioral Physiology, New York State Psychiatric Institute, New York, NY 10032 **(109)**

Justin M. Joffe, Department of Psychology, University of Vermont, Burlington, VT 05405 **(49)**

Theodore M. King, Department of Gynecology and Obstetrics, The Johns Hopkins University School of Medicine, Baltimore MD 21205 **(83)**

Michael T. Mennuti, Department of Obstetrics and Gynecology and Department of Human Genetics, University of Pennsylvania, Philadelphia, PA 19104 **(41)**

Heino F. L. Meyer-Bahlburg, Department of Psychiatry, College of Physicians and Surgeons of Columbia University and New York State Psychiatric Institute, New York, NY 10032 **(93)**

Allen A. Mitchell, Drug Epidemiology Unit, Boston University School of Medicine, Cambridge, MA 02138 (1)

Godfrey P. Oakley, Jr., Chief, Birth Defects Branch, Chronic Diseases Division, Bureau of Epidemiology, Center for Disease Control, Atlanta, GA 30333 **(33)**

The boldface number in parentheses following each contributor's affiliation is the first page of that contributor's chapter.

Ronald L. Poland, Department of Pediatrics, Wayne State University School of Medicine and Children's Hospital of Michigan, Detroit, MI 48201 **(129)**

Richard H. Schwarz, Professor and Chairman, Department of Obstetrics and Gynecology, State University of New York Downstate Medical Center, Brooklyn, NY 11203 **(xi, 153)**

Samuel Shapiro, Drug Epidemiology Unit, Boston University School of Medicine, Cambridge, MA 02138 **(1)**

Dennis Slone, Drug Epidemiology Unit, Boston University School of Medicine, Cambridge, MA 02138 **(1)**

Lester F. Soyka, Department of Obstetrics and Gynecology and Department of Human Genetics, University of Vermont College of Medicine, Burlington, VT 05405 **(49)**

Frank Witter, Department of Gynecology and Obstetrics, The Johns Hopkins University, School of Medicine, Baltimore, MD 21205 **(83)**

Sumner J. Yaffe, Professor of Pediatrics and Pharmacology, University of Pennsylvania and Children's Hospital, Philadelphia, PA 19104 **(xi, 157)**

Preface

On May 21 and 22, 1979 a symposium was held in New York on the subject of Drug and Chemical Risks to the Fetus and Newborn. The purpose of the symposium was to provide health professionals with the most current information about the impact of drugs and environmental chemicals upon the newborn. A group of international authorities was brought together to discuss both the acute and long term effects of these agents, not only when administered prenatally, but also by exposure through breast milk. It is hoped that this meeting and the published proceedings will stimulate investigation into the mechanism of drug and chemical effects and in that way contribute to the prevention of birth defects.

Richard H. Schwarz, MD
Sumner J. Yaffe, MD

Strategies for Studying the Effects of the Antenatal Chemical Environment on the Fetus

Dennis Slone, MD, Samuel Shapiro, MB, FRCP(E), and Allen A. Mitchell, MD

It is a remarkable fact that prior to 1941 little credibility was given to the notion that environmental factors might cause malformations to develop in the human embryo. This point of view was forcibly changed by Gregg's [1] classical demonstration in that year that rubella infection in the mother was teratogenic to the fetus. Since that time we have come to appreciate that many environmental factors of different kinds can adversely affect the fetus. Nevertheless, according to Wilson's estimates [2], the cause of fully 65% of malformations is still unknown, while some 25% may be due to genetic and chromosomal factors and about 10% to known environmental factors.

During the years since thalidomide was shown to be teratogenic, we have become increasingly sensitive to the multitude of potential hazards that the environment poses for the unborn child. In fact, biologists generally agree now that the human embryo is susceptible to many outside factors and that the maternal environment does not confer absolute protection against all adverse influences. Indeed, our concern about the potential adverse impact of environmental factors now extends beyond the zygote to effects mediated via the gametes prior to conception and to substances that might influence the mother's health and, in turn, affect the conceptus.

There is, however, a gap between these general principles, however valid they may be as biological philosophy, and the establishment of a practical approach with which to address the problems that confront our society; there is a demonstrated need to develop those strategies required to protect the fetus from the dangers posed by the chemical environment in which we live.

To quote McCann and Ames [3], "We are living in a sea of chemicals that have not been tested for their ability to cause cancer or birth defects." This metaphor is meant to be taken as all-encompassing and should serve to broaden our concern about a wide range of substances that are not generally thought of as potentially harmful to the fetus. Aside from drugs, which constitute the most

Drug and Chemical Risks to the Fetus and Newborn: 1–7

obvious and likely source for new teratogens, society must take measures to protect itself from the possible adverse effects of chemicals associated with our "life-style," such as alcohol, tobacco, cosmetics, and beverages; and also, we must pay greater attention to the growing number of chemicals that are an inevitable consequence of technology. These substances form part of our everyday environment at work, at home, while eating, drinking, and breathing. An extensive description of the range of chemicals involved has been published [4] and is redundant in this presentation.

In recent months, as though to provide emphasis to our concern about protecting the fetus from potential teratogens, we have witnessed the unfolding scandal of chemical waste disposal in the United States. A preliminary assessment by the Environment Protection Agency (EPA) [5] estimates that there are 32,000 sites that may contain hazardous wastes and that the number of sites that might contain significant quantities is 838. According to the EPA [6] some 35 million metric tons of industrial waste judged to be hazardous are produced annually in the USA. About 80% of this material is currently disposed of in ponds, lagoons, or landfills that are considered "non-secure." Thus it is not surprising that of the 50 industrial waste sites evaluated by the EPA in 1977, 86% showed migrations of hazardous chemicals into the groundwater [7]. Considering the magnitude of the waste disposal problem, it is chilling to consider that of the 60,000 chemicals in commercial use in the United States today, only 3,500 have been tested for teratogenicity in warm-blooded animals. Furthermore, between 1,500 and 2,000 chemicals are developed annually and introduced into our environment. What the long-term consequences of this problem are going to be in terms of the public health in general and embryogenesis in particular remains an open question.

It is now some 23 years since Minamata mercury disease was described in Japan [8], 19 years since the thalidomide disaster, and nine years since the discovery that diethylstilbestrol use during pregnancy [9] could cause clear cell cancer of the vagina in the female offspring. Even if these disasters could not have been foreseen, they would at least have been attenuated in terms of their magnitude by earlier recognition that preventable malformations were occurring. Moreover, since there have already been three major disasters attributable to the chemical environment in which we live, we cannot make the complacent assumption that there will be no problems in the future. Indeed, it is both possible and likely that unrecognized human teratogens are extant in our environment right now.

With these considerations in mind, the case for having comprehensive systems of surveillance devoted to the earliest possible detection of human teratogens would seen to be unarguable. Various systems exist, but they are insufficient for the need. Let us consider them briefly.

Worldwide, there are five programs that are national in scope, all in Europe [10]. An additional 12 or so programs operate on a regional basis, six of them in the United States. Of these, the largest monitors the hospital discharge records of approximately one million births annually, with the objective of detecting changes in rates of various malformations. This system is a collaborative effort involving the Department of Health, Education and Welfare, the Commission on Professional Health Activities, and the National Foundation – March of Dimes. This study is directed by the Birth Defects Branch of the Center for Disease Control in Atlanta. Two similar but smaller programs exist in Nebraska and Florida.

There are two other regional systems in the United States that not only register malformed infants but also collect interview data from mothers, including detailed histories of antenatal drug use and information about maternal occupation and place of residence.

Finally, there is one study that monitors spontaneous abortions. This study collects extensive interview data concerning exposure to various factors such as drugs, cigarettes, and alcohol, prior to and after conception.

The latter three systems are multipurpose in nature in that they are designed not only to test known hypotheses concerning possible teratogens but also to detect possible teratogenic agents as candidates for more detailed evaluation. To appreciate fully the potential utility of these studies, it should be noted that they can employ multiple comparisons with a view to identifying previously unsuspected associations. Conventional registries, on the other hand, permit the mounting of ad hoc studies, but they have no capability for discovery, other than the detection of changes in rates. The multipurpose studies also represent a departure from the conventional epidemiologic study, which is concerned solely with testing a specific hypothesis.

To sum up, although there have been interesting developments, the existing studies are not comprehensive enough to provide adequate public health surveillance for potential teratogens. At best, they constitute an incomplete system.

I would now like to turn to the elements required to develop a coherent and comprehensive strategy for preventing chemically induced damage to the fetus. In theoretical terms, the overall approach should, on the one hand, provide for the conduct of experiments to elucidate mechanisms and seek information on the effects of chemicals upon animals, tissue cultures, and bacteria. It is self-evident that experimental teratology has a central and vital role to play in identifying potential teratogens. Support for this branch of science should be adequate, long-term, and stable. In fact, it might be a good idea to consider the establishment of separate departments of teratology as a means of insulating this important research activity from the vagaries of a fluctuating biomedical research budget.

On the other hand, a variety of studies of human populations must be undertaken. There is little doubt that epidemiologic research methods have been successful in identifying etiologic factors for various cancers and many chronic diseases. These include cigarette smoking, asbestos, lead, and various drugs. There is no reason why these approaches should not be applied to the domain of teratology.

In our view, the full weight of these methods, expanded considerably both in concept and application, must be brought to bear on the problem posed by potential embryotoxins.

The implementation of such a strategy requires that an overall organizational framework be constructed to permit the development of the appropriate programs. We believe that the key ingredient for ensuring success is to organize a consortium of interests that would provide direction and stable financial support for a long-term effort in this field. By its very nature, research in this area requires the active support of the government, private foundations, industry, and the medical community.

Notwithstanding broad support from multiple sources, the government must assume the lead role for initiating, developing, and maintaining a program within the current health research establishment, whether it be in the National Institutes of Health or in some other agency. It will not be sufficient simply to provide additional funding. Rather, what is called for is an extramural program of directed research, supported and coordinated by a "center for teratology" within the appropriate federal setting. In fact, a model for this putative organization exists within the National Institute of Child Health and Human Development and is known as the Center for Population Research. It is characterized by coordinating an extensive program based upon perceived needs related to population research. Often when such a need is perceived a study will be initiated by the Center's own staff, which usually uses the contract mechanism to sponsor and fund the research.

An almost obligatory counterpart to any expanded effort in this field will require specially trained manpower. Thus, within any overall planning we should ensure sufficient postdoctoral training to provide for the application of experimental and epidemiologic methods to the problems at hand.

Assuming that there is tacit agreement regarding leadership, funding, and training, we can turn to the problems of conducting studies in human populations and ask what strategies are appropriate.

First, we should undertake a careful review of the existing monitoring and epidemiologic programs in the United States with a view to maximizing their utility. Indeed, a specific effort should be organized to involve a wide range of epidemiologists, who in the past have not been recruited to help resolve these problems. For example, the Birth Defects Monitoring Program, based upon discharge records of some 1,200 participating hospitals in the United States, represents a unique resource for monitoring the rates of malformations over time and provides a registry of malformed infants for conducting ad hoc case-control studies as needed. The question arises as to whether this resource is being fully exploited.

In a similar spirit, the Metropolitan Atlanta Program, the ongoing registries in Nebraska and Florida, and the case-control study relating drugs and malformations being conducted from Boston should be reviewed critically for their potential contribution to a national system.

Second, we should be on the lookout for innovative alternative approaches that could be implemented on a wide scale. For example, virtually all of the monitoring and surveillance schemes that have been mounted since the mid-1960s have involved, in the main, visible serious malformations observed at birth; little attention has been devoted to the study of spontaneous abortions. It is probable that the birth defects we observe reflect only the "tip of the iceberg" of human embryotoxicity. The first and the most ubiquitous effects of compounds that have teratogenic effects might thus be fetal loss. Therefore, a very sensitive indicator of environmental chemical effects on the fetus might very well be a system designed to monitor the rate of fetal wastage. Research workers at the Columbia University School of Public Health [11] have already suggested and published methods indicating that surveillance of spontaneous abortions is likely to be a powerful method of detecting environmental teratogens. They make the valid point that spontaneous abortions serve as a natural filtering device for the rejection of conceptuses with chromosomal and morphologic anomalies. It follows that a teratogenic agent that causes anomalies will, as a rule, produce an increased incidence of spontaneous abortions as well as an increased proportion of anomalous fetuses among the abortuses. This approach, which has been published by Kline and co-workers [12], represents a departure that appears to have great promise and certainly warrants careful review for its potential contribution and possible wide application.

Third, we should encourage studies in human populations that have as a principal objective the identification of teratogens and that rely upon a formal epidemiologic design. The appropriate model for these new studies would either be the current Metropolitan Atlanta system, the Boston study, or some version of the Finnish Malformation Registry [13]. Setting up such studies would not only result in producing higher quality data on birth defects, but would also promote the development of a research infrastructure with the experienced scientific staff needed to sustain epidemiologic studies in the field.

Finally, we should not forget the potential role that prepaid health care delivery systems could play in helping to identify environmental toxins. They have the virtue of providing a framework in which complete data on pregnancy outcome are available. Furthermore, in principle, information on drug consumption, lifestyle habits, and occupational exposure data from both parents are obtainable prior to knowledge of birth outcome, which minimizes potential bias in the reporting of such information. These inherent characteristics of health maintenance organizations make them particularly attractive as a framework upon which to construct teratologic studies.

In conclusion, let us remember that almost 20 years after the thalidomide disaster our defenses against similar chemically induced epidemics are meager; our knowledge of basic mechanisms of teratology, though growing, is insufficient; and in our view most important, formal epidemiological systems to detect early signs of chemically induced embryotoxicity are rudimentary. We have been fortunate that no major disaster appears to have occurred in recent years. However, we should not continue to trust in good fortune, but rather have the foresight to move to protect the fetus from a menacing chemical environment. It goes without saying that this objective will not be achieved either rapidly or without considerable cost.

It is important to remember that the fundamental issues with which we must deal in embryotoxicity and teratology are not isolated; rather they are manifestations of a much larger environmental crisis that we face in the public health domain. It is now apparent that much of the illness existing in contemporary society is either the consequence of our life-style habits such as cigarette smoking, or, frequently, the result of biological reaction to various insults such as mercury contamination of food. Birth defects due to teratogens have a special poignancy – they cause suffering to the most innocent of the innocent.

In planning for strategies to minimize the risk of abnormal embryogenesis, we have a responsibility to weigh our options carefully and make deliberate choices. No less than decisive action is called for to improve the odds in favor of normal fetal development in the biological lottery of human reproduction.

ACKNOWLEDGMENTS

This work was supported by contract 223-76-3016 from the Food and Drug Administration, contract N01-HD-6-2849 from the National Institute of Child Health and Human Development and contracts N01-CP-71029 and N01-CB-74099 from the National Cancer Institute, and a grand in aid from Hoffman-LaRoche, Inc.

The authors with to express their gratitude to Jacquelyn Smith, BSN, for her invaluable assistance in preparing the material for this paper.

REFERENCES

1. Gregg NM: Congenital cataract following german measles in the mother. Trans Ophthalmol Soc Aust 3:35, 1941.
2. Wilson JG: "Environment and Birth Defects." New York: Academic Press, 1973, p 49.
3. McCann J, Ames BN: A simple method for detecting environmental carcinogens as mutagens. In Saffiotti, Wagoner (eds): "Occupational Carcinogenesis." New York: Ann NY Acad Sci, 1976.

4. Wilson JG: Environmental chemicals. In Wilson JG, Fraser FC (eds): "Handbook of Teratology, Vol I. General Principles and Etiology." New York: Academic Press, 1977, p 360.
5. Preliminary assessment of clean-up costs for national hazardous waste problems. EPA publication, contract 68-01-5063, 1979.
6. Pierce C (ed): Hazardous waste fact sheet. EPA Journal 5:12, 1979.
7. "Solid Waste Facts, A Statistical Handbook." U.S. Environmental Protection Agency, # SW-694, August 1978.
8. Tsubaki T, Irukayama K (eds): "Minamata Disease." New York: North-Holland, 1976, p 3.
9. Herbst AL, Scully RE: Adenocarcinoma of the vagina in adolescence: A report of seven cases including six clear cell carcinomas (so-called mesonephromas). Cancer 25: 745, 1970.
10. Flynt JW, Hay J: International clearinghouse for birth defects monitoring systems. In Klingberg MA, Wetheral JAC (eds): "Epidemiological Methods for Detection of Teratogens." Basel: S. Karger, 1979, p 44.
11. Stein Z, Susser M, Warburton D, Wittes J, Kline J: Spontaneous abortion as a screening device. Am J Epidemiol 102:275, 1977.
12. Kline J, Stein Z, Strobino B, Susser M, Warburton D: Surveillance of spontaneous abortions. Am J Epidemiol 106:345, 1977.
13. Saxen L, Klemetti A, Haro AS: A matched pair register for studies of selected congenital defects. Am J Epidemiol 100:297, 1974.

Critical Periods of Prenatal Toxic Insults

Allen S. Goldman, MD

Genetic and/or environmental insults to the developing child within the womb have been classically considered either as killing the embryo or producing congenital malformations during the critical first trimester. Congenital malformations have been defined as structural abnormalities present at birth. These concepts have been considerably changed or amplified by several principles of prenatal toxicity that have been derived from observations made during the past two decades (Table I). In this chapter the effects of a variety of environmental agents that are known or are suspected to be toxic to human development will be traced from the development of the eggs and sperm to lactation to illustrate these principles. For this purpose teratogenic (malforming) agents will be defined as those that produce (at a critical period of development) an abnormal presence, absence, or quantity of a substance or agent that is required for, or can interfere with, the developmental program.

TABLE I. Principles of Teratogenesis and Timing of Toxicity

1. The kind of effect a genetic and/or environmental toxic insult produces depends upon the time in development at which it acts.
2. A toxic agent may affect the embryo even when given prior to conception either to the mother or to the father.
3. The same toxic agent may disrupt the developmental program and produce a congenital malformation at one time but only injure an organ at another.
4. A toxic agent may also produce defects at different levels of biologic organization resulting in biochemical, physiological, or behavioral malformations that may not be apparent at birth.
5. Toxic agents may be devastating to the embryo but harmless to the mother.
6. The earlier in the formation of a structure a toxic agent acts, the more complete is the damage to that structure.
7. Susceptibility to embryotoxicity depends upon the genotype of the embryo and the manner in which the agent interacts with the genotype.

Drug and Chemical Risks to the Fetus and Newborn: 9–31

Perhaps the most important principle is that the kind of effect a genetic and/or environmental toxic influence produces depends upon the time in development at which it acts. This principle is depicted schematically in Figure 1. The figure presents a summary of the timing of embryo-toxic or fetotoxic agents, possible effects, and possible maternal factors that may influence the degree and nature of the fetal effects.

DEVELOPMENT OF GAMETES

Development of Eggs

The first period depicted in Figure 1 is that of the development of the egg and the sperm. The length of time involved in the development of the egg is vastily different from that of the sperm. The development of the human egg begins in the ovary of the mother, while she, herself, is a fetus. At this develop-

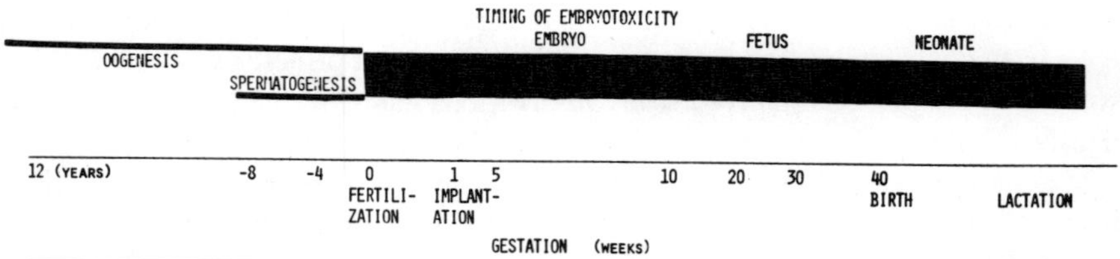

	HORMONES	PHENYTOIN	HORMONES	METHYLMERCURY	TETRACYCLINES	I.V. FLUID	DIAZEPAM
	LSD	THALIDOMIDE	CONTRACEPTIVES	DIETHYLSTIBESTROL	QUININE	PITRESSIN	LITHIUM
	?	METHADONE	ABORTIFACIENTS	THALIDOMIDE	CHLOROQUINE	SALICYLATES	HEXACHLOROBENZENE
		ESTROGEN	?	PHENYTOIN	GOITROGENS	VITAMIN K	METHYLMERCURY
				TRIMETHADIONE	THIOURACIL	NAPHTHALENE	SULFONAMIDES
				ALCOHOL	TERIDAX	GANGLIONIC	ATROPINE
DRUGS				WARFARIN	SALICYLATES	BLOCKERS	ANTICOAGULANTS
				AMINOPTERIN	HEAVY METALS	RESERPINE	ANTITHYROIDS
				ESTROGEN	ANTIBIOTICS	MORPHINE	ANTIMETABOLITES
				ANDROGEN	SMOKING	SEDATIVES	CATHARTICS
				PROGESTIN		ANALGESICS	DIHYDROTACHYSTEROL
				AMINOGLUTETHIMIDE		AMMONIUM	IODIDES
						CHLORIDE	NARCOTICS
						CARDIOVASCU-	TETRACYCLINES
						LAR DRUGS	METRONIDAZOLE
MICROORGANISMS				RUBELLA	RUBELLA		HERPES
				TOXOPLASMOSIS	TOXOPLASMOSIS		CYTOMEGALOVIRUS
				VARICELLA	VARICELLA		VARICELLA
				SYPHILIS	SYPHILIS		
				CYTOMEGALOVIRUS	CYTOMEGALOVIRUS		
				HERPES	HERPES		
RADIATION	X-RADIATION			ATOMIC RADIATION			
	CHROMOSOMAL	DEATH	PREMATURITY	PREMATURITY	PREMATURITY	NEONATAL	INFANT
POSSIBLE	DAMAGE	ABORTION	ABORTION	ABORTION	ABORTION	MORBIDITY	MORBIDITY
EFFECTS	?	MALFORMATION		DEATH	ORGAN DAMAGE		
	DEATH	PREMATURITY		MALFORMATION	FETAL MORBIDITY		
	AGE		NEURAL	NUTRITION	MATERNAL DISEASE	MATERNAL	
	?		ENDOCRINE	MATERNAL DISEASE	?	DISEASE	
MATERNAL	SEASON		STATE	CROWDING		?	
FACTORS	METABOLISM			SOCIAL CLASS			
	EMOTIONS			GEOGRAPHY			
				SEASON			

Fig. 1. Drugs and modifying maternal factors reported to have toxic effects on the embryo or fetus and critical periods of human development.

mental stage all of the mother's eggs will enter the first division of meiosis. Meiosis is the unique process of cell division that reduces the number of chromosomes from 46 to 23. A single replication of the chromosomes followed by two consecutive cell divisions halves the number of chromosomes. The union of egg and sperm at fertilization restores the number of chromosomes to 46. However, ova are arrested in late prophase of the first meiotic division until just before ovulation. In some oocytes this may not occur until 45 or more years after birth. Such a long delay may account in part for the relatively high frequency of meiotic nondisjunction. This time period also may explain why environmental agents have been so difficult to detect as potential causes of chromosomal damage.

Development of Sperm

Spermatogonia, which have been dormant in the seminiferous tubules of the testis since the fetal period, begin to increase in number at puberty. After several mitotic divisions the spermatogonia grow and undergo gradual changes that transform them into primary spermatocytes, the largest germ cells in the tubules. Each primary spermatocyte subsequently undergoes the first division of meiosis to form two secondary spermatocytes. These secondary spermatocytes undergo a second meiotic division to form four spermatids, which are gradually transformed into four mature sperms. This process of transformation of an immature germ cell into a mature sperm, including meiosis, takes about 64 days.

Insults During Development of Gametes

The kind of effect produced by toxic agents during the period of gametogenesis is death of the sperm or egg, chromosomal defects, or embryonic death leading to early abortion. Chromosomal breaks have been found in meiotic cells after high doses of LSD in mice [1]. Somatic cells of nine children exposed in utero to LSD showed a significant increase in chromosomal breakage, but there were no associated abnormalities [2]. In a prospective study of 972 children, a significantly greater number of trisomics was found after maternal abdominal radiation exposure [3].

One study reported twice the expected rate of children with Down syndrome after maternal treatment with ovulation-inducing agents (clomiphene citrate and menotropins) [4]. At any rate, whatever genetic or environmental factors may be operative during gametogenesis, they produce their effects in the ovary during the time the mother develops from a fetus to within two to three days after ovulation, and in the testis, up to 64 days prior to conception.

The Father and Congenital Malformations

Two reports in the 1960s concerned the birth of a defective child whose father only had taken thalidomide [5]. Moreover, malformed rabbit fetuses have been produced by giving thalidomide only to their fathers prior to conception [6]. These observations suggested that paternally derived teratogenicity may be due to the presence of drugs in semen, which may adversely affect fertility or produce congenital malformations either directly or through the sperm. Thalidomide and/or thalidomide metabolites have been found in rabbit semen after administering ^{14}C-thalidomide to male rabbits [7]. Thalidomide added to the semen in vitro became bound to the rabbit spermatozoa [7]. Similarly, male rats that are given methadone [8, 9] or caffeine [10] generate offspring with low birthweights and diminished neonatal survival. Methadone is excreted in high concentrations into semen of man [9] and of rabbits [9]. It has been long known that birth defects occur more frequently in mothers who have epilepsy and are under anticonvulsant treatment with diphenylhydantoin [11]. It has also been suggested recently that offspring of epileptic fathers who are under anticonvulsant treatment may be defective when born of normal mothers [12]. Recently, diphenylhydantoin has been shown to be present in human and rabbit semen [13]. Thus, it is possible that some drugs may affect human development through the semen.

EARLY EMBRYONIC DEVELOPMENT

Fertilization of the egg by the father's sperm occurs within 24 to 36 hours after ovulation (Fig. 1). The dividing morula converts into a blastocyst during the next three or four days while passing down the fallopian tube, and the late blastocyst implants in the uterus of the human about the sixth or seventh day. During the remainder of the second week after conception the extraembryonic membranes are laid down, the embryonic disc is formed, and the process of gastrulation or development of the three germ layers occurs during the third week. Thus, by the time the first menstrual period is missed the embryo is in the primitive streak stage.

Insults in the Early Embryonic Period

The period of early embryonic development, which occupies the first three weeks of pregnancy, has been generally thought to be relatively insensitive to embryotoxic influences, primarily because of the failure of most experimental agents to affect early embryonic development when administered to pregnant animals. However, it is possible to interfere with blastocyst formation in rabbits both in vitro and in vivo by drugs [14]. During this period the most probable effect is severe damage and death of the embryo with subsequent abortion. There is an increased incidence of abnormalities in aborted embryos and fetuses [15]. An example of an active teratogen at this time is the antihypercholesterolemic drug, triparanol, now withdrawn from use, which is an active teratogen in rats when given as early as day 4 prior to implantation [16]. This drug, or its active constituent, requires some time to be activated. Other drugs acting at this time include actinomycin D [17], cyclophosphamide [18], and cyanoketone [19]. In the case of actinomycin D, interference with early differentiation could be caused by DNA binding with corresponding blocking of RNA synthesis [20]. Implantation of the embryo has been prevented by maternal administration of estrogen. A number of chemicals and drugs have been shown to penetrate into tubular fluid and even into the preimplantation blastocyst when administered to pregnant rabbits in doses comparable to those encountered in the human [21]. Thus, this period may also prove to be a critical one.

EMBRYONIC PERIOD

Congenital Malformations

The embryonic period occurs between four and nine weeks of pregnancy and is the primary critical period for congential malformations. The available human data agreed upon by most authors indicate that the embryonic period is susceptible to a variety of environmental teratogenic influences (listed in Fig. 1) that are capable of disrupting the developmental program.

Complexity of the Developmental Program

What is a developmental program? The process of human development can be considered a series of genetically preprogrammed instructions carried in the structure of the DNA of the egg. These instructions regulate all of the biochemical transformations necessary to attain the chemical diversity of the adult at specified critical periods. The complexity of the human developmental program is a staggering 100 billion bits of information. This is calculated on the basis of the diversity of H, C, O, and N atoms in a cubic millimeter of the unfertilized egg [22] and on the basis of the diversity of the nucleotide pairs in the DNA in the human chromosomes [23]. A single letter of the alphabet is defined by six bits (binary digits), and the information content of a single page is 10,000 bits. Thus, the complexity of the program of human differentiation is equivalent to 10 million printed pages, or the contents of a huge library. The Viking landers that reached the surface of Mars in 1976 each had preprogrammed instructions of a few million bits – ie, the information content between that of a bacterium and an alga. Considering the enormous complexity of human differentiation, it is astonishing that errors in the developmental program are so few, amounting at most to less than 7% of births.

Toxic Insults and the Developmental Program

How do toxic insults interfere with the developmental program? They probably disrupt the preprogrammed instructions contained within the human zygote at critical periods of development. They probably do this by producing an abnormal amount of a substance (high or low) that either is required for or can interfere with the developmental program. Martians interested in learning how the Viking lander works might try to disrupt the preprogrammed instructions. If they did this with a sledgehammer, they would not learn as much as they could by stopping the program with "antibodies" to certain transistors. Unfortunately, almost all of our understanding of toxic insults known to affect human differentiation is of the "sledgehammer" variety.

However, some of the complexities of the program of the hormonal control of human sexual differentiation have been unraveled by studies that used specific natural and experimental fetal hormone-depriving agents as "antibody to transistor" types of probes [19]. The program of male differentiation appears to be directed by fetal testosterone through the same chain of molecular events by which testosterone produces its hormonal action in the adult. This molecular chain of events is initiated genetically at different critical periods. Gonadotropically stimulated testicular synthesis of testosterone makes a complex of androgen-receptor protein in the cytosol of various target organ cells. After incorporation into target organ nuclei the androgen-receptor complexes cause DNA- and RNA-directed synthesis of male specific proteins. Interference with this program at any of a variety of sites involving fetal testosterone either in its synthesis, circulation, or its uptake or action in the target organs allows the inborn female program to be expressed. This interference can be: antibodies to gonadotropins, inhibitors of specific testosterone biosynthetic enzymes, antibodies to testosterone, or antihormone blockers of the receptor protein; as well as genetic deficiencies of testosterone biosynthetic enzymes (congenital adrenal hyperplasia) or of androgen-receptor proteins (testicular feminization).

Table I shows a list of insults and Table II shows the drugs that most investigators agree are embryotoxic in humans. The criteria upon which Table II was based consist of agents that produce a higher percentage of developmental defects or intrauterine death in infants of women exposed to them compared to those of nonexposed women. In many of these cases animal models of the defects exist. Moreover, Table II contains those drugs that are also suspected to be embryotoxic in man, based on retrospective surveys indicating definite evidence of teratogenicity. Exposure to methyl mercury produces a serious set of malformations of the central nervous system becoming manifest at six months of age in congenital Minamata disease [24]. Thalidomide, perphaps the best known teratogen, produces malformations of several systems but most notably phocomelia [25]. Several cases of malformations of sexual differentiation have occurred after maternal administration of sex hormones [19, 26–28]. These hormones include estrogens, androgens, and progestins. Stilbestrol produces genital malformations of the male and female during the 4–12-week critical period fetus [19, 26, 29–33] and also produces transplacental carcinogenesis of the human vagina up to 18 weeks [30]. A characteristic fetal malformation syndrome has been recognized to be due to adminstration of folic acid synthesis

TABLE II. Embryotoxic Drugs in Man

Drug	Number of cases	Effect	References
Thalidomide	8,000	Thalidomide embryopathy Limbs, ears, eyes, internal organs	[25]
Hormones			
Androgens	37	Females – fusion of labia Clitoral hypertrophy (virilization)	[52]
Progestins	>600	Females – virilization	[42]
	9	Males – hypospadias (feminization)	[26–28]
Estrogens			
Diethylstilbestrol	4	Females – virilization	[29]
	>90%	Females – vaginal adenosis, cervical ridges	[30]
	>200	Females – postpubertal cervical clear cell carcinoma	[30]
	28	Males – hypospadias or meatal stenosis, deficient sperm	[31–33]
Progestins and estrogens	28	Males – behavior and personality	[55, 56]
Folic acid antagonists			
Aminopterin	17	Cranial dysostosis, craniofacial	
Amethopterin	1	anomalies, cleft palate, talipes	[34]
Alcohol	>60	Fetal alcohol syndrome – retardation, palpebral fissure shortening, craniofacial, limb	[35]
Anticonvulsants			
Phenytoin	51	Fetal hydantoin syndrome – craniofacial, limb, hypoplasia of phalanges and nails, growth defect	[37, 38]
Tridione	>16	Fetal tridione syndrome – craniofacial, cleft palate	[39]
Aminoglutethimide	3/5	Females – virilization	[40]
Anticoagulants			
Warfarin	14	Nasal hypoplasia – chondrodysplasia punctata: Conradi-Hünermann syndrome	[41]
Alkylating agents			
Chlorambucil	1/3	Agenesis, kidney and ureter	[40]
Busulfan	2/27	Cleft palate, eye, genitalia	[40]
Cyclophosphamide	2/5	Ectrodactyly, digit defects	[40]
Nitrogen mustard	2/7	Digital and renal defects	[40]
Iodides	39	Goiter, hypo- and hyperthyroidism	[40]
Propylthiouracil	18	Exophthalmos, goiter	[40]
Methimazole	2	Neonatal deaths	[40]
^{131}I	12	Thyroid ablation	[40]
Miscellaneous	32	Goiter	[40]

inhibitors, such as aminopterin, which were administered as abortifacients in women for whom a later surgical intervention was planned [34]. This has led to either lethal or teratogenic effects in their fetuses. Recently, several human fetal syndromes have been ascribed to other teratogens, which include the fetal alcohol syndrome [35, 36], fetal hydantoin syndrome due to phenytoin [37, 38], and the fetal trimethadione syndrome [39]. Sexual malformations of females have occurred after maternal administration of the cholesterol desmolase inhibitor, aminoglutethimide [40]. Several cases of infants with extreme hypoplasia of the nasal cartilage and stippling of the bones as a phenocopy of Conradi-Hünermann disease or chondrodysplasia punctata have been reported to be due to the fetal warfarin syndrome [41]. A few cases of various anomalies have been reported after the use of certain alkylating agents and of goitrogens.

Table III shows drugs that are possibly embryotoxic in man. These drugs produce questionable increases in defects or deaths among offspring of exposed women, based on large numbers of accumulated cases or on extensive epidemiologic surveys; or the drug has definite embryotoxic potential in more than one animal species, especially at high doses. There is increasing epidemiologic evidence that salicylates are associated with pregnancy wastage and are soft teratogens in children [42]. Salicylates produce defects in rats, mice, and rhesus monkeys [42]. In one report [43] of cleft palate 14.9% of mothers had taken salicylates compared to 5.6% of control mothers. Three surveys in different countries implicate diazepam as an oral clefting teratogen [44–46]. One study reported teratogenicity of chlordiazepoxide and meprobamate [47] but none was found in 1,870 pregnancies [48]. Several studies have indicated increased risk for malformation produced by antihistamines, especially meclizine, but several subsequent prospective studies failed to provide validation [57, 58]. Several retrospective reports have indicated the use of estrogen-progestin contraceptive drugs during early weeks of pregnancy as soft teratogens for congenital heart disease [42, 49]. This has also been confirmed in a large prospective study [50]. Congenital limb-reduction defects have been also reported in association with contraceptive drugs in one report [51] and a clustering of a syndrome-like occurrence of vertebral, cardiac, tracheal, esophageal, renal, and limb anomalies in another [49]. However, other studies have found no teratogenicity of these preparations [42]. Thus, one has to regard contraceptive preparations as possible teratogens. Many antibiotics are definitely teratogenic in rodents, but early reports of increased risk of human anomalies with various antibiotics were not confirmed, although one prospective study observed an excess of cleft (lip) palate in mothers taking penicillins and tetracyclines and/or chloramphenicol in the first trimester [43]. Deafness has been reported in 6/50 children exposed in utero to streptomycin [59] and in more than 50 children exposed to quinine [42]. Antitubercular drugs have also conflicting reports of teratogenicity, but some reports indicate increased teratogenicity [42]. Lithium salts used for psychotherapy are suspected to be

TABLE III. Possible Embryotoxic Drugs in Man

Drug	Number of cases	Effect	References
Salicylates	>144	Decreased birthweight, higher mortality, increased clefts, and eight cases of various malformations	[42]
Tranquilizers			
Diazepam	>64	Cleft palate	[43–46]
Chlordiazepoxide	11–12/100 versus	Various	[47]
Meprobamate	2–4/100	Heart defects	[47]
	0/1870	None	[48]
Antihistamines			
Benzylhydrylpiperazines	12/6124	Cleft palate	[57]
(meclizine, cyclizine)	600/31,000		[58]
Contraceptives			
Progestogen–estrogen	>108	Limb defects	[51]
	>119	Vertebral, anal, cardiac	[49]
	>32	Tracheal, esophageal, renal, limb	[49]
Anorexics			
Amphetamine	20	Heart	[40]
Antibiotics			
Streptomycin	6/50	Deafness	[59]
Penicillin, Tetracyclines/and/or chloramphenicol	9	Clefts	[59]
Antitubercular drugs	12/23	Various	[42]
Isoniazid	5/125	Cerebral dysfunction	[42]
Antimalarials			
Quinine	>50	Deafness and various	[42]
Insulin shock	2/14	Deaths	[40]
	4/14	Various	
Lithium carbonate	13/143	Various	[42]
Corticoid hormones	8/688	Cleft (lip) palate	[52, 53]
Caffeine	44/202 versus 21/192 >8 cups coffee/day	Various	[54]

a teratogen [42]. There is some evidence [52, 53] for oral clefting teratogenicity of maternal and synthetic adrenocortical hormones. Recently, evidence [54] for teratogenicity of caffeine has been presented. In this study women who drank more than eight cups of coffee a day had twice the number of malformations as did suitable controls. Amphetamines have also been linked to cardiac malformations in humans [40].

Most drugs that malform the fetus, such as anti-cancer drugs, also produce some side-effects that may lead to maternal illness. The thalidomide experience demonstrates, however, that the fetus may be greatly malformed by an agent that produces little to no adverse effect on the mother. This principle further complicates detection of malforming drugs.

Physiologic, Biochemical, or Behavioral Malformations

In the last two decades it has become apparent that a new kind of effect that agents may have on the unborn child is that of retarded or defective postnatal function or behavior without obvious anatomic defect. Studies in both women and men and laboratory animals have shown that prenatal administration of low doses of sex hormones, which may have no apparent effect on brain morphogenesis, produce long-term alterations in brain function [55, 56]. In general, the defects are a prevention of masculine behavior in males or induction of masculine behavior in females.

Maternal alcohol consumption results in retarded development, impaired learning capability, and a decreased reproductive potential without obvious anatomic defect [60]. The postnatal administration of morphine in animals has been reported to alter body weight gain, locomotor activity, neonatal mortality, tolerance to the analgesic effects of morphine in adulthood, eye opening activity in open field test, pubertal onset, and the adrenal stress response [61]. Moreover, the administration of D-amphetamine prenatally results in postnatal abnormalities in motor behavior and brain biogenic amine levels [62]. Consequently, this area of interest of postnatal biochemical and behavioral defect without obvious anatomic defect is an exciting area in the timing of malformations that should yield considerable information of value to human development.

FETAL PERIOD

The fetal period, extending from approximately eight or nine weeks of gestational age to birth is primarily a period of fetal growth (Fig. 1). The kind of fetal effect occurring during this period is prematurity, abortion, organ or tissue injury, and possibly malformation. Most studies show that infection with microorganisms during the first three months of pregnancy results in true organ malformations in the sense that they are disruptions of the developmental program [63]. However, when contracted after the first trimester to term, such infections may produce primarily organ damage, such as, the cases of congenital encephalitis occurring in mothers with Venezuelan equine encephalitis between 13 and 36 weeks [64]. This damage resulting at a later fetal stage may be regarded more as a type of tissue injury [63] rather than a malformation (which may result from any postnatal infection).

Quinine, and antimalarial no longer in common clinical use, sometimes produced near deafness in both children and their mothers [65]. Chloroquine has similar effects [40]. Tetracycline administered during this period is deposited in fetal bones where the antibiotic persists to inhibit markedly fetal and neonatal bone growth [65] and cause staining of the teeth [66]. At this time maternal treatment with antithyroid drugs, such as propylthiouracil, ^{131}I, etc, may produce goiter or hypothyroidism in the child [40]. Salicylates during this period have been associated with prematurity and abortion and fetal morbidity in a few cases of hemorrhagic pneumonia [42]. Heavy metals have been described to have fetotoxic effects [42]. Antibiotics also produce certain toxic effects in the fetus [42]. Smoking has been shown to cause reduced fetal birthweight and increased fetal morbidity [67]. However, true developmental defects also may be produced at this time, such as morphologic insults to the brain or functional defects that only become manifest postnatally [68].

Teridax was used about two decades ago for the visualization of the gallbladder [69]. The use of this contrast medium in pregnant mothers during this period gave rise to an abnormal elevation of protein-bound iodine from the normal newborn level of 4–5 mg/dl to 4,000–5,000 mg/dl. Since the administration of this material may have been up to as much as two years prior to the conception of the affected child, this observation illustrates the principle that the time of action of any agent may long postdate the time of its administration.

Birth

Figure 1 lists a variety of agents that produce harmful effects in the newborn child when administered to the mother just before birth or during the often overlooked period of breast feeding [70].

MATERNAL FACTORS

Figure 1 lists the timing of several maternal factors that may either be directly embryotoxic or fetotoxic or that may indirectly influence susceptibility of the embryo or fetus to malformation or damage by several agents.

Nutrition

The effects of general malnutrition were studied in human populations under severe conditions of famine, such as occurred during World War II [71]. Amenorrhea and irregularity of menstrual cycles were common, leading to a marked decrease in the birth rate. For infants conceived during famine, the incidence of abortions, stillbirths, neonatal deaths, and malformations were all higher than for pre-war births. In more recent clinical investigations, cardiovascular abnormalities [72] and retarded development of postnatal bone growth [73] were seen in infants malnourished before birth. About 10% of infants with fetal growth retardation had physiological problems postnatally that resulted from congenital anomalies. A clinical study was carried out in Montreal in which the mothers were given nutrition education [74]. If the women had poor nutrition, nutritional supplements were provided. The incidence of stillbirths, perinatal mortality, and neonatal mortality was lower in the group with improved nutrition than in Quebec or Canada as a whole.

Maternal Disease

An interesting possible cause of athyrotic cretinism was suggested when a 25% incidence of thyroid antibodies was observed in mothers giving birth to athyrotic infants [75]. Whether the antibodies crossed the placenta and ablated the fetal thyroid with the secondary result of maternal and fetal thyroid damage has not been determined. Congenital hyperthyroidism associated with deafness and mental retardation is commonly found in offspring of goitrous mothers residing for long periods in iodine-deficient areas. Treatment of maternal hyperthyroidism with antithyroid agents may produce goiter or hypothyroidism in the child after the beginning of function of the fetal thyroid during the fourth month of gestation [59].

Masculinization of the external genitalia of the female fetus occurs in pregnant women with masculinizing tumors, which include arrhenoblastomas, adrenal arrest, luteoma, and Leydig cell, Brenner, and Krukenberg tumors. The source of the virilization is androgens of tumor origin, and if the androgens are produced before nine weeks of gestation, a completely masculinized penile urethra results in the female [19]. Otherwise, if the androgens are produced after this time, only clitoral hyperthrophy may result.

Infants of diabetic mothers have a higher incidence of congenital anomalies, in general, and of the caudal regression syndrome (agenesis or hyperplasia of the femurs and agenesis of the lower vertebrae), in particular [76]. Although improved prenatal diabetic management and neonatal care has reduced fetal wastage and death from respiratory disease, the incidence of congenital malformations has now replaced respiratory distress syndrome as the most common cause of death of infants of diabetic mothers [77]. The defects in the diabetic embryopathy occur prior to the seventh week of pregnancy [78].

Embryotoxicity has also been reported with severe maternal hypoglycemia and in mothers with toxemia of pregnancy. These factors, however, are not well understood.

Emotional Stress

The ancient belief that severe maternal psychogenic factors, such as, fright, shock, or stress may lead to malformations has largely been discounted in this century. However, in the last few years several animal investigations have suggested a renewed look at this question in light of disturbed maternal endocrine or autonomic functions. Electric stimuli to the maternal hypothalamus in rabbits or exposure to increased noise in pregnant rats or mice at critical periods leads to malformations. The production of anomalies in rats by salicylate poisoning is enhanced by maternal immobilization, crowding, or isolation to the degree that anomalies are produced by low, otherwise nonteratogenic, doses of salicylate [79]. This immobilization effect can be prevented by a sedative, sodium phenobarbital, or a tranquilizer, chlorpromazine [80]. Thus, the immobilization effect illustrates another principle of timing of malformations – that the state of the mother may alter susceptibility to teratogenic agents.

Various malformations and anomalies were also induced in fetuses of mice parabiotically stressed on the sixth, seventh, or eight day of pregnancy and in fetuses of crowded pregnant mice [81]. The hypothesis that the teratogenic and other effects were consequences of prolonged prenatal maternal stress induced by the experimental conditions is supported by the observation that both procedures led in a short time to significant increases in maternal adrenal weight.

Social Class

Markedly higher incidences of anomalies of the central nervous system along with mental deficiency have been reported to occur in lower social classes in studies performed in Britain and North America [82]. The reasons for this association are not clear but probably include environmental and possibly genetic factors.

Geography and Season

The incidence of anencephaly varies among certain Europenas, Asians, and Africans [82]. There are geographic differences in the rates of spina bifida between north and south of the United States and in cleft palate between Hawaii and Wisconsion or New Jersey. Higher levels of background radioactivity have been observed in areas having higher frequencies of anomalies, such as in the southwestern United States and certain areas of New York. Seasonal variation in rates of congenital malformations has been found in studies of England, Japan, Canada, and Ohio [82]. The reasons for these associations again are not clear.

Ethnic Variation

There is evidence that prevalence of neural tube defects in the descendants of immigrants tends to move from the levels associated with their ancestral home towards those found in other residents of their places of birth [82]. Thus, the

Japanese of Hawaii have an incidence of spina bifida well above the low levels occurring in Japan, although not as high as that in the Caucasians of Hawaii. Similarly, in the descendants of immigrants from the regions of high prevalence in the British Isles to places of lower prevalence, anencephaly and spina bifida seem to be less common than in the regions of their ancestors, although higher than that of their neighbors. This tendency of a prevalence shift of immigrants towards that of their neighbors appears to be gradual and is more marked in grandchildren and remoter descendants of the immigrants.

CRITICAL PERIODS OF TERATOGENICITY

Thalidomide

Figures 2–5 depict in schematic form the expanded development of several organ systems [83–85], with timing of specific malformations due to thalidomide derived from several authors [86–89]. Malformations resulting from incomplete morphogenesis usually have their origin prior to the time the organ structure is

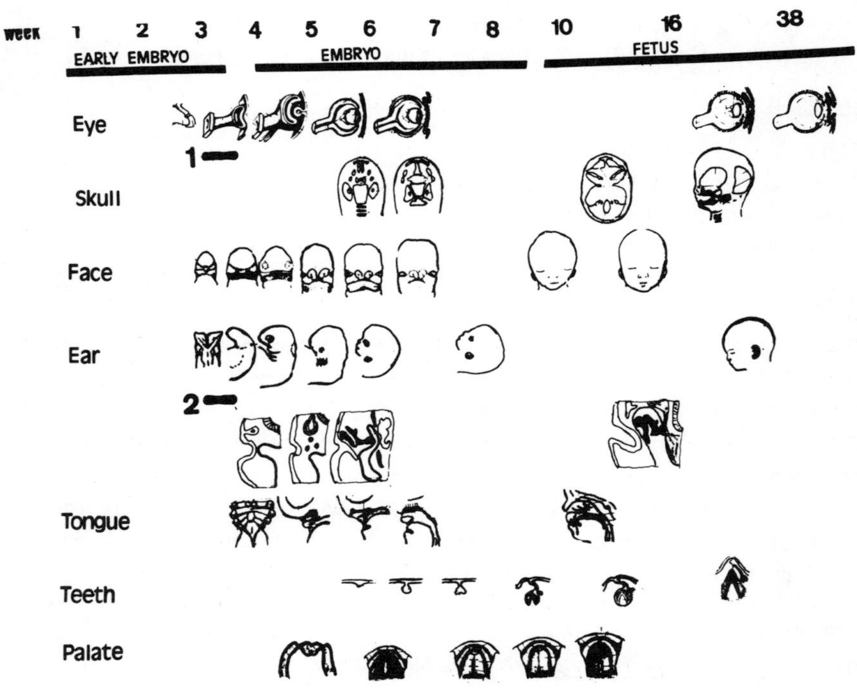

Fig. 2. Expanded embryonic period and timing of thalidomide-induced malformations. Specific defects: line 1, anophthalmia, microphthalmia; line 2, anotia.

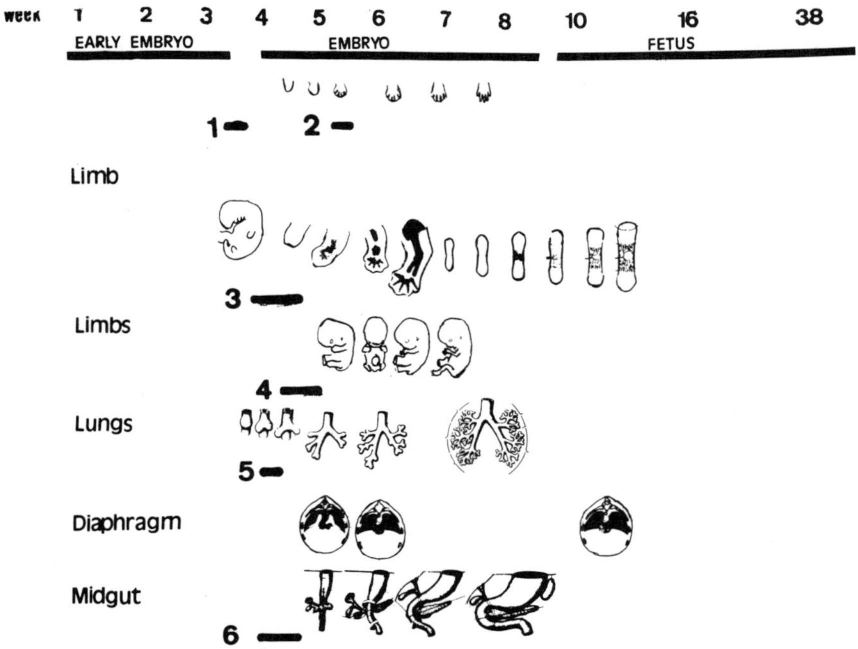

Fig. 3. Expanded embryonic period and timing of thalidomide-induced malformations. Specific defects: line 1, duplication of thumbs; line 2, triphalangism of thumbs; line 3, phocomelia, amelia of arms; line 4, phocomelia of legs; line 5, pulmonic lobe agenesis; and line 6, duodenal and gallbladder atresia.

completed. One cannot generally say that a developmental defect occurred at this particular time; all that one can say is that the problem existed prior to this particular time. However, the thalidomide experience allowed a precise correlation with occurrence of various developmental anomalies in children with the start of maternal exposure. Thus, a timetable of thalidomide effects on various organs can be constructed.

Figure 2 shows the critical period of certain craniofacial development. The timing of maternal administration of thalidomide is 20–24 days after conception, when eye defects (anophthalmia and coloboma) (line 1) and ear defects (microtia, anotia) (line 2) resulted. Thus, thalidomide appears to disrupt completely or partially eye and ear development at the formation of the optic cup and optic placode.

Figure 3 illustrates the developmental staging of the limb and certain viscera. Duplication of the thumbs is produced during the formation of the limb bud at 20–24 days after conception (line 1); triphalangism of thumbs during the separa-

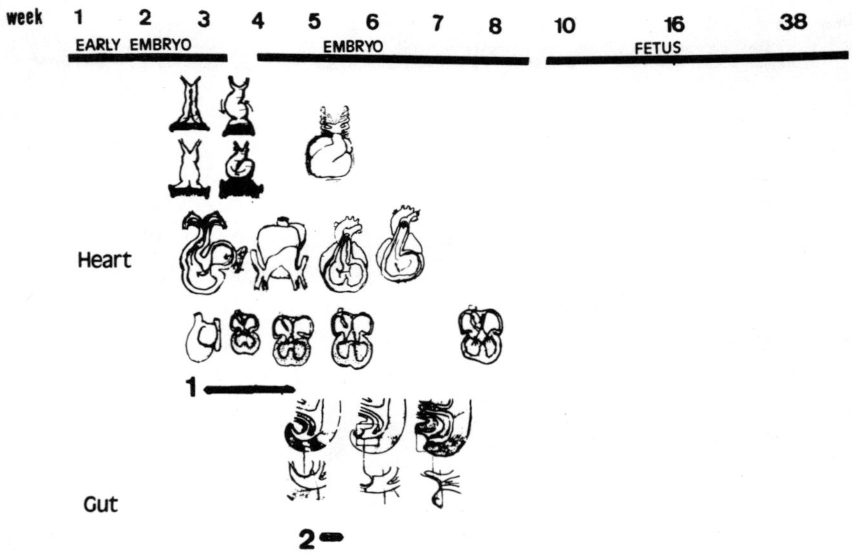

Fig. 4. Expanded embryonic period and timing of thalidomide-induced malformations. Specific defects: line 1, heart and vessel anomalies; line 2, rectal stenosis.

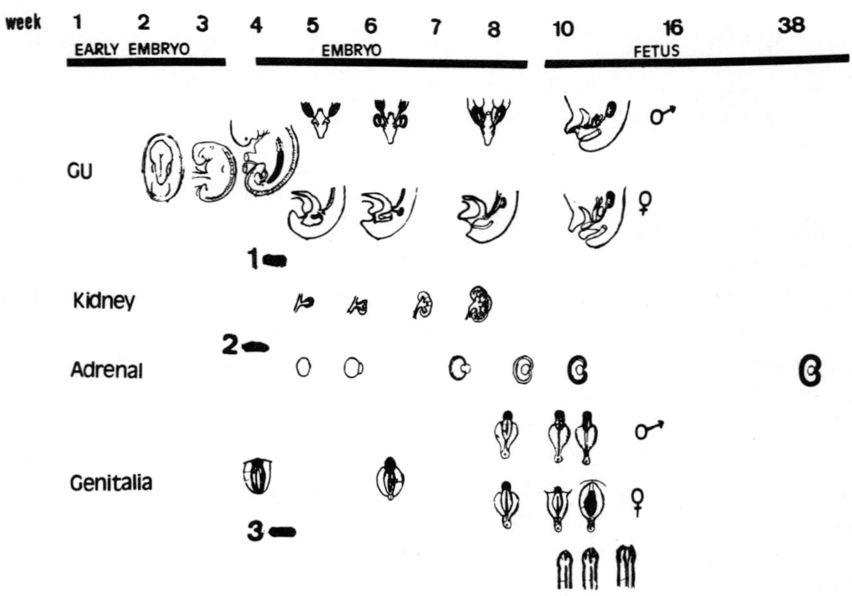

Fig. 5. Expanded embryonic period and timing of thalidomide-induced malformations. Specific defects: line 1, urogenital sinus; line 2, renal agenesis; line 3, genital defects (urogenital sinus).

tion of the digital rays 34–35 days (line 2); phocomelia of the arms at 24–33 days during the formation of the arm buds (line 3); phocomelia of the legs at 28–33 days during the formation of the leg buds (line 4); agenesis of pulmonary lobes at 27–29 days during the formation of the pulmonary lobes (line 5); and duodenal and gallbladder atresia at 26–31 days during the earliest formation of these structures (line 6).

Figure 4 shows the timing of certain aspects of cardiovascular and gastrointestinal development. The timing of thalidomide administration is 22–33 days after conception for the occurrence of the heart and vessel defects (line 1) and 35–36 days for rectal stenosis (line 2).

Figure 5 shows the timing of urogenital development. Urogenital defects (urogenital sinus) occur when thalidomide is taken 27–29 days after conception (lines 1 and 2) and renal anomalies (agenesis) at 24 days (line 2).

Rubella

Figure 6 shows the frequency of abnormalities in 108 offspring related to time of maternal rubella infection. The majority of developmental defects are

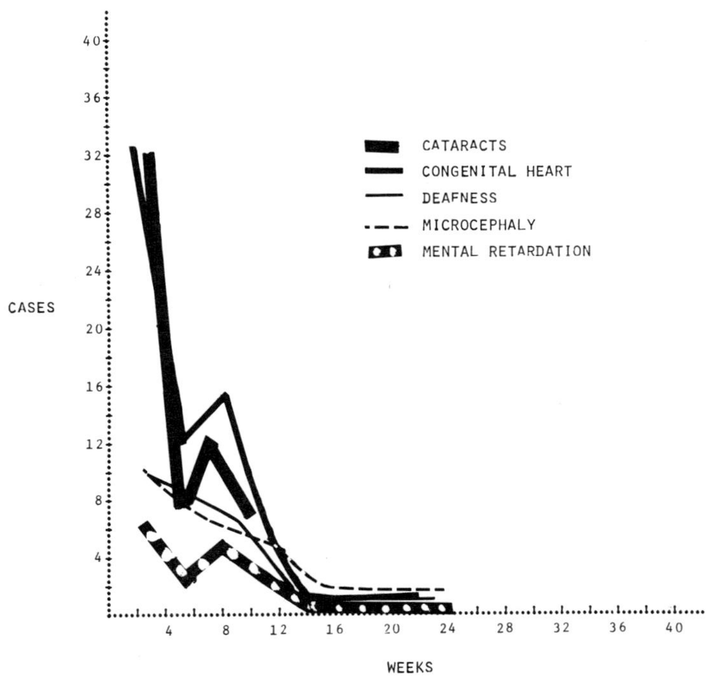

Fig. 6. Frequency of abnormalities in offspring related to time of maternal infection with rubella [data from reference 63].

produced by rubella when maternal infection was contracted in the first month (50%) or second month (22%); however, only 6–8% of infants are malformed when maternal infection occurs in the third to fifth months [63]. Thus, it can be seen that the critical period of embryonic teratogenic vulnerability to rubella virus is quite similar to that of thalidomide.

VALUE OF TIMING

It is almost self-evident that the ability to correct developmental defects will depend upon a fundamental understanding of the timing and mechanism of the defects. The nature of external genital defects occurring in congenital adrenal hyperplasia and of the malformations of sexual differentiation produced by maternal administration of sex hormones has been explained by an understanding of the mechanism and timing of the different defects occurring in the two sexes. This understanding allowed for the precise correction of these defects in exact experimental animal models of these diseases [19].

Our early work in the area of congenital sexual malformations in man uncovered the fact that, in addition to the well-known virilizing effects of progestins and estrogens, these agents also produced feminization of males, manifested mainly by hypospadias [19, 26]. We pointed out that these effects were probably produced by inhibition of fetal 3β-hydroxysteroid dehydrogenase by these agents

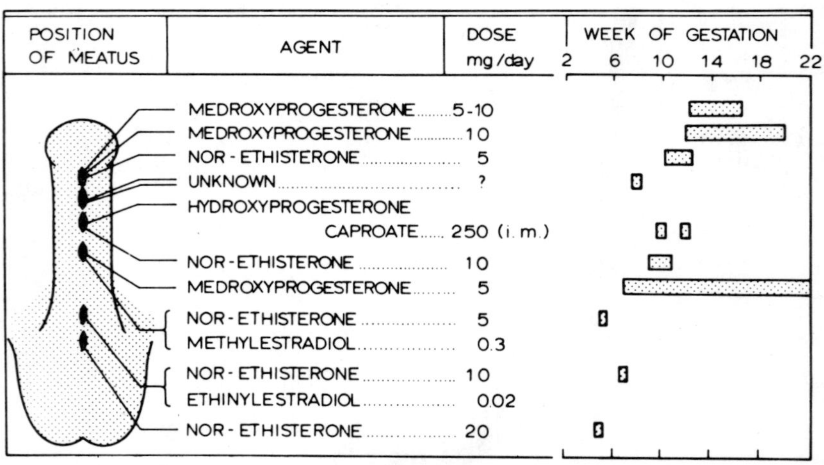

Fig. 7. Six cases of hypospadias in male offspring related to time of beginning of maternal treatment with various estrogens and progestins. Note that the closer the time of treatment to beginning of penis formation the more severe the hypospadias [data from reference 28].

in a manner similar to the occurrence of these defects in human congenital adrenal hyperplasia due to a genetic deficiency of this enzyme [26]. Moreover, we pointed out that the closer to the time of penis formation that the mother took the progestins, the more severe the degree of hypospadias [26]. This timing was confirmed by Aarskog (Fig. 7) [27, 28]. These warnings led to the withdrawal of hormonal pregnancy test drugs from the market in Norway in 1970, and their use has recently been discontinued in the United Kingdom [28].

Another example of the potential usefulness of an understanding of the timing of malformations is our recent observation that the congenital malformations that are significantly more common in infants of diabetic mothers must occur prior to the seventh gestational week [78]. This makes the often postulated cause of the defects, insulin, unlikely as the teratogenic mechanism, since the human fetus is not exposed to fetal or maternal insulin during this period. Thus, if one hopes that the improvement in prenatal diabetic management, which has reduced fetal wastage and death, will reduce malformations, this management will have to be instituted during the first seven weeks of pregnancy.

DIAGNOSTIC PRINCIPLES OF TIMING

An evaluation of any particular patient from a developmental point of view should include a validation of the abnormalities. In some cases this may lead to more precise timing by measurement when possible. For example, if there is a defect in palatal closure involving only the posterior portion, then the time prior to which this defect must have occurred can be more precisely determined as between the beginning of palatal closure during the ninth week to the completion of fusion during the twelfth week. The timing should be proportional to the amount of fusion that has occurred.

In a patient with multiple malformations the concepts of anomalad and syndrome [85] are useful. The term "anomalad" has been suggested to denote that a cluster of anomalies may result from a single earlier defect, whereas the term "syndrome" connotes multiple malformations in one or more tissues that are not explained by a single localized early defect in morphogenesis. On this basis the Pierre-Robin anomalad would result from early mandibular hypoplasia before the eight to ninth week. Thus, it behooves those physicians who see newborns to describe as carefully as possible those malformations that constitute a syndrome or an anomalad to permit more accurate timing of the defect.

In conclusion, the point of this paper is to illustrate principles of malformations derived from the consideration of timing and to present a summarized list of human teratogens and their timing for the physician to consider and avoid. It is hoped that this goal has been accomplished and that areas of potential interest have been indicated.

ACKNOWLEDGMENTS

This research was supported in part by grants DE-4622 and DE-5041 from the National Institutes of Health and from The National Foundation – March of Dimes.

REFERENCES

1. Skakkebaek NE, Philip J, Rafaelson DJ: LSD in mice: Abnormalities in meiotic chromosomes. Science 160:1246, 1968.
2. Cohen MM, Hirschhorn K, Verbo S, Frosch WA, Groeschel MM: The effects of LSD-25 on the chromosomes of children exposed in utero. Pediatr Res 2:486, 1968.
3. Uchida IA, Holunga R, Lawler C: Maternal radiation and chromosomal observations. Lancet 2:1045, 1968.
4. Oakley GP, Flynt JW: Increased prevalence of Down's syndrome (mongolism) among the offspring of women treated with ovulation-inducing agents. Teratology 5:264, 1972.
5. Editorial: The drugged sperm. Br Med J 1:1063, 1964.
6. Lutwak-Mann C: Observations of progeny of thalidomide-treated male rabbits. Br Med J 1:1090, 1964.
7. Lutwak-Mann C, Schmid K, Keberle H: Thalidomide in rabbit semen. Nature 214:1018, 1967.
8. Smith DJ, Joffe JM: Increased neonatal mortality in offspring of male rats treated with methadone or morphine before mating. Nature 253:202, 1975.
9. Joffe JM, Peterson JM, Smith DJ, Soyka LF: Sub-lethal effects on offspring of male rats treated with methadone before mating. Res Commun Chem Pathol Pharmacol 13:611, 1976.
10. Soyka LF, Joffe JM, Peterson JM, Smith SM: Reduction in perinatal survival of caffeine treated male rats. Pediatr Res 12:409, 1978.
11. Meadow SR: Anticonvulsant drugs and congenital abnormalities. Lancet 2:1296, 1968.
12. Shapiro S, Hartz SC, Siskind V, Mithcell AA, Slone D, Rosenberg L, Monson RR, Heinonen OP: Anticonvulsants and parental epilepsy in the development of birth defects. Lancet 1:272, 1976.
13. Swanson BN, Leger RM, Gordon WP, Synn RK, Gerber N: Excretion of phenytoin into semen of rabbits and man. Drug Metab Disposition 6:70, 1978.
14. Lutwak-Mann C, Hay MF: Effect on the early embryo of agents administered to the mother. Br Med J 2:944, 1966.
15. Nishimura H, Takano K, Tanimura T, Yosuda M: Normal and abnormal development of human embryos: First Report of the analysis of 1,213 intact embryos. Teratology 1:281, 1968.
16. Roux C: Action teratogene du triparanol chez l'animal. Arch Fr Pediatr 21:451, 1964.
17. Wilson JG: Effects of acute and chronic treatment with actinomycin D on pregnancy and the fetus in the rat. Harper Hosp Bull 24:109, 1966.
18. Brock N, Kreybig T von: Experimental data on testing of drugs for teratogenicity in laboratory rats. Naunyn Schmiedebergs Arch Pharmacol 249:117, 1964.
19. Goldman AS: Abnormal organogenesis in the reproductive system. In Wilson JG, Fraser FC (eds): "Handbook of Teratology," Vol. II, New York: Plenum Press, 1977, pp 391–421.
20. Wilson JG: Embryologic considerations in teratology. Ann NY Acad Sci 123:129, 1965.

21. Fabro S, Sieber SM: The foeto-placental unit. In Pecile A, Finzi C (eds): "International Congress Series No 183" Amsterdam: Excerpta Medica 1969, p 313.
22. Dancoff SM, Quastler H: The information content and error rate of living things. In Quastler H (ed): "Essays on Information Theory in Biology." Urbana, Illinois: University of Illinois Press, 1953.
23. Britten RJ, Davidson EH: Gene regulation for higher cells: A Theory. Science 165: 349, 1969.
24. Weiss B, Doherty RA: Methylmercury poisoning. Teratology 12:311, 1975.
25. McBride WG: Thalidomide embryopathy. Teratology 16:79, 1977.
26. Goldman AS, Bongiovanni AM: Induced genital anomalies. Ann NY Acad Sci 142:755, 1967.
27. Aarskog D: Clinical and cytogenetic studies in hypospadias. Acta Paediatr Scand Suppl 303:1, 1970.
28. Aarskog D: Current concepts in cancer: Maternal progestins as a possible cause of hypospadias. N Engl J Med 300:75, 1979.
29. Bongiovanni AM, DiGeorge AM, Grumbach MM: Masculinzation of the female infant associated with estrogen therapy alone during gestation. J Clin Endocrinol Metab 19: 1004, 1959.
30. Herbst AL, Scully RE, Robboy SJ, Welch WR: Complications of estrogen use – Prenatal therapy with diethylstilbestrol. Pediatrics 62(Suppl):1087, 1978.
31. Henderson BE, Benton B, Cosgrove M, Baptista J, Aldrich J, Townsend D, Hart W, Mack TM: Urogenital tract anomalies in sons of women treated with diethylstilbestrol. Pediatrics 58:505, 1976.
32. Kaplan N: Male pseudohermaphrodism. N Engl J Med 261:641, 1959.
33. Bibbo M, Gill W, Azzizi F et al: Follow up study of male and female offspring of DES exposed mothers. Obstet Gynecol 49:1, 1977.
34. Warkany J: Aminopterin and methotrexate: Folic acid deficiency. Teratology 17: 353, 1978.
35. Mulvihill JJ, Yeager AM: Fetal alcohol syndrome. Teratology 13:345, 1976.
36. Clarren SK, Smith DW: The fetal alcohol syndrome. N Engl J Med 298:1063, 1978.
37. Hanson JW: Fetal hydantoin syndrome. Teratology 13:185, 1976.
38. Weber M, Schweitzer M, Mur JM, Andre M, Tridon P, Vert P: Epilepsie, medicamentes antieleptiques et grossesse. Arch Fr Pediatr 34:374–383, 1977.
39. Goldman AS, Yaffe SJ: Fetal trimethadione syndrome. Teratology 17:103, 1978.
40. Schardein JL: "Drugs as Teratogens." Cleveland: CRC Press, 1976.
41. Warkany J: Warfarin embryopathy. Teratology 14:205, 1976.
42. Wilson JG: Embryotoxicity of drugs in man. In Wilson JG, Fraser FC (eds): "Handbook of Teratology," Vol. I New York: Plenum Press, 1977, p 309.
43. Saxen I: Associations between oral clefts and drugs taken during pregnancy. Int J Epidemiol 4:37, 1975.
44. Safra MJ, Oakley GP: Association between cleft lip with or without cleft palate and prenatal exposure to diazepam. Lancet 2:478, 1975.
45. Saxen I, Saxen L: Association between maternal intake of diazepam and oral clefts. Lancet 2:498, 1975.
46. Aarskog D: Association between maternal intake of diazepam and oral cleft. Lancet 2:921, 1975.
47. Milkovitch L, van den Berg BJ: Effects of prenatal meprobamate and chlordiazepoxide hydrochloride on human fetal embryonic and fetal development. N Engl J Med 291:1268, 1974.
48. Hartz SC, Heinonen OP, Shapiro S, Siskind V, Slone D: Antenatal exposure to

meprobamate and chlordiazepoxide in relations to malformations, mental development, and childhood mortality. N Engl J Med 292:726, 1975.
49. Nora JJ, Nora A, Blu J, Ingram J, Fountain A, Peterson M, Lortscher RH, Kimberling WJ: Exogenous progestogen and estrogen implicated in birth defects. JAMA 240: 837, 1978.
50. Heinonen OP, Slone D, Shapiro S: "Birth Defects and Drugs in Pregnancy." Littleton Massachusetts: Publishing Science Group, 1977.
51. Janerich D, Piper JM, Glebatis DM: Oral contraceptives and congenital limb-reduction defects. N Engl J Med 291:697, 1974.
52. Serment H, Ruf H: Les dangers pour le produit de conception de medicaments administrés à la femme enceinte. Bull Fed Soc Gynecol Obstet Lang Fr 20:69, 1968.
53. Fraser FC: Pregnancy and adrenocorticoid hormones. Br Med J 2:479, 1962.
54. Borlée I, LeChat MF, Bouckaert A, Misson C: Le Café, facteur de risque pendant la grossesse? Louvain Med 97:279, 1978.
55. Yalom I, Greene R, Fisk N: Prenatal exposure to female hormones: Effect on psychosexual development in boys. Arch Gen Psychiatry 28:554, 1973.
56. Reinisch J: Prenatal exposure of human fetuses to synthetic progestin and oestrogen affects personality. Nature 266:561, 1977.
57. Lenz W: How can the teratogenic action of a factor be established in man? South Med J 64(Suppl 1):41, 1971.
58. Sadusk JF, Palmisano PA: Teratogenic effect of meclizine, cyclizine, and chlorcyclizine. JAMA 194:987, 1965.
59. Shepard TH: "Catalog of Teratogenic Agents." Baltimore: Johns Hopkins University Press, 1976, p 208.
60. Streissguth AP: Maternal alcoholism and the outcome of pregnancy: A review of the fetal alcohol syndrome in alcoholism, problems in women and children. In Greenblatt M, Schuckit MA (eds): "Seminars in Psychiatry." New York: Grune & Stratton, 1976, p 251.
61. Zimmerman E, Sonderegger T, Bromley B: Development and adult pituitary adrenal function in female rats injected with morphine during different postnatal periods. Life Sci 20:639, 1977.
62. Hitzeman BA, Hitzeman RJ, Brase DA, Loh HH: Influence of prenatal d-amphetamine on development and behavior of rats. Life Sci 18:605, 1976.
63. Kurent JE, Sever JL: Infectious diseases. In Wilson JC, Fraser FC (eds):"Handbook of Teratology," Vol I. New York: Plenum Press, 1977, p 225.
64. Wenger F: Venezuelan equine encephalitis. Teratology 16:359, 1977.
65. Cohlan SQ, Bevelander G, Tiamsic T: Growth inhibition of prematures receiving tetracycline: A clinical and laboratory investigation of tetracycline-induced bone fluorescence. Am J Dis Child 105:353, 1963.
66. Cohlan SQ: Tetracycline staining of teeth. Teratology 15:127, 1977.
67. Meyer MB: How does maternal smoking affect birth weight and maternal weight gain. Am J Obstet Gynecol 131:888, 1978.
68. Rodier PM: Correlations between prenatally-induced alterations in CNS cell populations and postnatal function. Teratology 16:235, 1977.
69. Lucey JF: Hazards to the newborn infant from drugs administered to the mother. Pediatr Clin North Am 8:413, 1961.
70. Hervada AR, Feit E, Sagraves R: Drugs in breast milk. Perinatal Care 2:19, 1978.
71. Smith CA: Effects of maternal under nutrition upon the newborn infant in Holland (1944-1945). J Pediatr 30:229, 1947.

72. Naeye RL, Diener MM, Dellinger WS: Urban poverty: Effects on prenatal nutrition. Science 166:1026, 1969.
73. Wilson MG, Meyers HI, Peters AH: Postnatal bone growth of infants with fetal growth retardation. Pediatrics 40:213, 1967.
74. Primrose T, Higgins A: A study in human antepartum nutrition. J Reprod Med 7:257, 1971.
75. Chandler RW, Blizzard RM, Hung W, Kyle M: Incidence of thyrocytotoxic factor and other anti-thyroid antibodies in the mothers of cretins. N Engl J Med 267:376, 1962.
76. Gabbe SG: Congenital malformations in infants of diabetic mothers. Obstet Gynecol Surv 32:125, 1977.
77. Soler NG: Perinatal medicine. Stockholm, 5th European Congress of Perinatology. 1976, p 108.
78. Mills JL, Baker L, Goldman AS: Malformations in infants of diabetic mothers occur before the seventh gestation week: Implications for therapy. Diabetes 1979 (in press).
79. Goldman AS, Yakovac WC: The enhancement of salicylate teratogenicity by maternal immobilization in the rat. Pharmacol Exp Ther 142:351, 1963.
80. Goldman AS, Yakovac WC: Prevention of salicylate teratogenicity in immobilized rats by certain central nervous system depressants. Proc Soc Exp Biol Med 115:693, 1964.
81. Hamburgh M, Rader LM, Lang A, Silverstein H, Hoffman K: Malformations induced in offspring of crowded and parabiotically stressed mice. Teratology 10:31, 1974.
82. Leck I: Correlations of malformation frequency with environmental and genetic attributes in man. In Wilson JG, Fraser FC (eds): "Handbook of Teratology," Vol I. New York: Plenum Press, 1977, p 243.
83. Nishimura H, Shiota K: Summary of comparative embryology and teratology. In Wilson JG, Fraser FC (eds): "Handbook of Teratology," Vol. III. New York: Plenum Press, 1977, p 119.
84. Moore K: "The Developing Human," Ed 2. Philadelphia: WB Saunders, 1977.
85. Smith DW: "Recognizable Patterns of Human Malformation: Genetic, Embryologic and Clinical Aspects." Philadelphia: WB Saunders, 1976.
86. Kreipe V: Missbildungen innerer Oragane bei Thalidomidembryopathil. Arch Kinderheilkd 176:33, 1967.
87. Lenz W: Chemicals and malformations in man. In Fishbein M (ed): "Second International Conference on Congenital Malformations." New York: International Medical Congress, Ltd., 1964, p 263.
88. Lenz W: Ein Vergleich der sensiblen Phase fuer Thalidomid im Tierversuch und beim Menschen. Arch Kinderheilkd 177:259, 1968.
89. Lenz W: The susceptible period for thalidomide malformations in man and monkey. Ger Med Aron 13:197, 1968.

Causal Inference in Teratology

Godfrey P. Oakley, Jr., MD, MSPH

A recurring theme in medical school was that medicine is both an art and a science. In recent years, it has been stressed that medicine is more science than art. Certainly, as a medical student I was primarily impressed with the science. Thalidomide embryopathy was discovered then, and I accepted the causal relationship. Furthermore, I assumed that drugs in general were known either to be safe or unsafe. Unfortunately, I later learned that for most drugs and environmental agents there are few systematically collected and analyzed human data from which to draw teratogenic inferences. Such judgments are, therefore, more art than science. This morning I would like to explore the art and science of causal inference. In taking illustrations from historial data, there will be opportunity for me to appear to be "Monday morning quarterbacking," which is not my intention. Since causal inference is not totally science, there must be judgments; some of these, both positive and negative, will be wrong. The question is whether we can learn to reduce the errors in judgment.

Susser has pointed out that there are three main approaches to making causal inferences: the population or epidemiology approach, the case approach, and the experimental laboratory approach. I will discuss only the population and case approaches [1].

POPULATION APPROACH TO CAUSAL INFERENCES

The most respected approach to causal inference is the clinical trial. In this population approach, subjects are randomly assigned to a treatment or nontreat-

The opinions expressed in this article are those of the author and not necessarily those of the Department of Health, Education and Welfare.

Drug and Chemical Risks to the Fetus and Newborn: 33–39

ment situation, and the change in a disease process is observed to see if it differs between the two groups. This methodology has been extremely helpful in delineating whether a drug is efficacious. Because of its success with efficacy, there is a prevalent opinion among some medical scientists that a study that is not prospective like a clinical trial is hardly worth doing and cannot be relied upon. Such a judgment considerably underplays the value of other approaches. There are qualitative differences among approaches, but they can all contribute pertinent data. Even the clinical trial itself is no paragon. Well-financed and well-executed trials can give results upon which it is difficult to base a decision for or against a given treatment. If you doubt this conclusion, I would suggest you recall the controversy concerning the danger and efficacy of oral anti-diabetic agents that still exists in light of the UGDP Study.

Clinical trials per se have not been very useful for making causal inferences regarding teratogenic and other adverse effects. There are two reasons. First, one does not deliberately set out to show that a drug is bad; rather, that it is good. Furthermore, there is a sample size problem. Since all members of a trial are sick, the opportunity to see improvement from therapy is relatively good and might be shown on a sample size, for instance, of 100 to 300 patients. Such a sample size is so small, however, that one could miss quite a real increase in an adverse effect such as a birth defect. For example, if in such a small study a new drug caused a fivefold increase in the incidence of anencephaly, a 1/1,000 disease, there would be little chance of detecting such an increase. The diethylstilbestrol (DES) adenocarcinoma of the vagina story is an excellent example to show how the sample-size problem is real and why it is poor judgment to require "prospective" or clinical-trial data before making a causal inference. The long-term follow-up of the clinical trials of DES have failed so far to turn up a single case of adenocarcinoma of the vagina. Rather than disproving a causal relationship, these negative studies only tell us that the adverse effect was a relatively uncommon event even after exposure.

Clinical trials are one kind of cohort study. In epidemiologic evaluation of environmental agents a different kind of cohort or prospective study is done. In these studies, a group of exposed and a group of unexposed individuals are identified. The frequency of an adverse outcome is then measured in the two groups. This kind of study differs from the clinical trial in that persons are not randomly allocated to exposed and unexposed groups. Such studies have played a major role in making causal inferences about cancer. In studies of the adverse health effect of cigarette smoking, for example, there were two major cohort studies. In one, the smoking habits of British physicians were defined and the incidence of cancer was determined among smokers and nonsmokers. In this country, the American Cancer Society used volunteer workers to enlist friends in a similar type of study. Such cohort studies have seldom played a major role in identifying human teratogens because of the sample size problem mentioned for the clinical trials and because they are very expensive studies to do. Such expensive studies would usually only be done to test a hypothesis of a causal relationship of a major teratologic public health problem. As Dr. Slone mentioned, there simply have not been resources devoted to such costly epidemiologic studies of birth defects.

The more common epidemiologic method is the case-control one. Here, a group of people with an adverse effect is selected, along with a comparison group without the adverse outcome. The frequency of exposure to a putative teratogenic agent is determined in the case and control groups. For example, the DES story was brought to light based upon only eight cases and 32 controls [2]. The association with DES was so striking that causality seemed quite probable.

Monitoring the incidence of a disease over time is another epidemiologic technique. Changes in incidence, either increases or decreases, are usually observed in the absence of a hypothesis. It then becomes necessary to do more definitive studies to try to elucidate the cause of the change in incidence. For example, in the Birth Defects Monitoring Program in recent years, we have seen substantial increases in patent ductus arteriosus, ventricular septal defects, and renal agenesis [3]. We are unaware of the causes of these increases. To be considered with biologic causes are changes in reporting habits and diagnostic habits of physicians.

CASE APPROACH TO CAUSAL INFERENCE

Let us move from the population methods to the case methods. The case method has also been referred to as the alert practitioner method. Here, it is the striking unusualness of the clinical manifestations and/or the exposure that suggests a causal relationship. Such one-by-one observations seldom prove causality. They have often, however, played a major role in identifying the correct hypothesis for which a causal relationship was established through formal case control and/or cohort studies. What are the limitations of such observations? First, even in those situations in which causality can be inferred, how often malformations occur and to what degree after what exposure cannot be known. Furthermore, the possibility of false-positive associations is high. If one questions a group of mothers of malformed babies, it is easy to identify for each mother several first-trimester exposures to drug and other environmental agents. A multitude of hypotheses, therefore, can be generated, the majority of which would be false-positive. The number of reported false-positive hypotheses is kept down by the fact that clinicians seldom think that there are any striking peculiarities. Because of thalidomide, there seems to be a bias toward case reports related to structural abnormalities of the limbs. The case method also suffers false-negative observations. For example, the fetal alcohol syndrome association was passed over by clinicians and epidemiologists alike for centuries.

CAUSAL INFERENCES IN TERATOLOGY

Thalidomide

Thalidomide was suspected of being a teratogenic agent by two different clinicians (Dr. Lenz in Germany and Dr. McBride in Australia). In making the causal inference they used both case-control and cohort methods. Dr. Lenz used a case-control method, as he had seen about 50 cases and determined that all of the mothers gave a history of having taken thalidomide; whereas in about 300 women who had had normal babies, none gave a similar history [4]. Dr. McBride's experience came from a clinical trial of morning sickness in his hospital. About nine months after the beginning of that trial he had ascertained some malformed babies and was suspicious that the drug caused their deformities. When the study was about 18 months old he was even more suspicious [5]. There were nearly simultaneous publications in *The Lancet* describing these studies. A causal relationship was highly likely based on those data and was finally established with additional studies.

Alcohol

The fetal alcohol syndrome was first reported from this country by Jones, Smith, Ulleland, and Streissguth [6]. The methodologies involved a combination of the alert practitioner approach and the cohort approach. Dr. Ulleland had been following infants of alcoholics for some time and had selected from them a group that she was concerned about. Jones and Smith, the dysmorphologists, viewed eight of these children, all of whom had been exposed to high levels of alcohol in utero, and they depicted a pattern of defects among four. Based on similar clinical observations, a causal inference between a pattern of birth defects and a history of severe maternal alcoholism is generally accepted. There remain many questions, however, about the relationship. Is it something other than alcohol in common with severe alcoholism that causes the problem? If it is alcohol, at what dose does the problem begin, what manifestations of the adverse fetal effect occur at what doses, for what length of exposure, and at what times during gestation? Answers to these questions simply are not available. In the absence of hard data, it has been recommended that pregnant women not have more than two drinks a day.

Tridione

Tridione became a suspected teratogen based on the work of a geneticist, J. German, and his colleagues [7]. In studying family histories of congenital heart disease they encountered two families in which it appeared that the use of Tridione in pregnancy was related to a high probability of adverse outcome (either spontaneous abortion or congenital heart disease). Further reported cases have similar facies and the presence of severe congenital heart disease [8]. Thus, one can conclude, based on case studies, that Tridione is teratogenic. It is not possible, however, to know how often this syndrome occurs at varying doses and differing gestational times of exposure.

Lithium

Lithium is a drug that is used to treat depressive psychoses. Its use is relatively rare. J.J. Nora, a pediatric cardiologist, became suspicious that it was a teratogen when he observed two children with a rare cardiac defect, Ebstein anomaly, whose mothers had taken lithium [9]. He then approached a lithium registry that had been maintained for several years by different investigators and discovered that six of 118 babies that had been reported to that registry had cardiac defects; two of them had Ebstein anomaly and one had tricuspid atresia. I believe it reasonable, based on these kinds of clinical case data, to conclude that lithium is a human teratogen. The exact risk, however, remains to be defined.

Diazepam

Diazepam is a widely sold tranquilizer. Suspicions about this drug arose from two case-control studies. One was a case-control study conducted in Finland by Saxen and Saxen who found about a twofold relative risk between exposure and isolated cleft palate and cleft lip with or without cleft palate [10]. In a smaller case-control study Safra and Oakley noted an approximately fourfold relative risk between isolated cleft lip with or without cleft palate [11]. No secular trends were noted. One positive and one negative study have since been reported. There have been no one-by-one case reports to impugn the drug. Such case reports seem unlikely, because both the defect and exposure are relatively common. It is likely the final answer will have to be resolved by extensive epidemiologic studies. At present one can only say that a suspicion has been raised. Certainly, one cannot conclude, based on present evidence, that the drug is a teratogen.

CONCLUSION

For the vast majority of drugs there is even less teratologic information available than has been presented for the few drugs listed here. As our society has become more concerned about adverse environmental agents, the package labeling of drugs has changed. For example, the Physicians Desk Reference (PDR) used to say that a drug was not known to be harmful where there was little if any human data. Now, with virtually the same information on a drug, the PDR would say that the drug is not known to be safe. The restatement is of value in reducing drug exposure in pregnancy. It is not very helpful, however, when one has to counsel a pregnant patient contemplating abortion who has been exposed to a drug for which there is very little information. She needs some quantitative measure. Fortunately, Heinonen and associates have examined the relationship between birth defects and drug usage among the participants in the Collaborative Perinatal Study and have published their findings in a book [12]. A clinician can use that book to see what the experience with a drug was in that study and can usually give some quantitative risk. The catalogue of Shepard and his review article also are useful to physicians faced with a drug exposure during pregnancy for which there is little information available [13, 14]. Many times the drug will have been marketed for years without an indication of teratogenicity, yet no systematic search has been made. The absence of suspicion does not mean the drug is without teratogenic properties. My rule of thumb in such instances is that if a teratogenic risk exists, it is unlikely that the risk would exceed twice the background risk.

With present-day concerns about drugs and environmental agents as teratogens, we must try to place the information in perspective. If we do not, it is possible that there will be a large number of "unnecessary" abortions. Such a practice was so common after diagnostic radiation that the American College of Radiologists has produced a statement indicating the low magnitude of risk after diagnostic radiation [15].

The raison d'être for concern about drugs and chemicals causing birth defects is prevention. Excluding alcohol, the number of infants born each year with birth defects known to be caused by drugs and chemicals is small. In contrast, there are 5,000 infants born each year with anencephaly or spina bifida. Maternal serum alpha-fetoprotein screening could reduce by 4,000 the number of infants born each year with these two common and serious birth defects. It is essential to be ever searching for drug and chemical causes of birth defects; however, we must realize that, with drugs, a considerable search has occurred over the last 20 years with little impact on birth defect incidence. It would be a serious error if the search for drug and chemical teratogens were given priority over the development and implementation of new techniques of prenatal diagnosis.

REFERENCES

1. Susser M: "Causal Thinking in the Health Sciences." New York: Oxford University Press, 1973.
2. Herbst AL, Ulfelder H, Poskanzer, DC: Adenocarcinoma of the vagina. N Engl J Med 284:878–881, 1971.
3. Center for Disease Control: Congenital Malformations Surveillance Report. April 1977–March 1978, Issued November 1978.
4. Lenz W: Thalidomide and congenital abnormalities. Lancet 1:45, 1961.
5. McBride WG: Thalidomide and congenital abnormalities. Lancet 2:1358, 1961.
6. Jones KL, Smith DW, Ulleland CN, Streissguth AP: Pattern of malformations in offspring of chronic alcoholic mothers. Lancet 1:1267–1271, 1973.
7. German J, Ehlers KH, Kowal A, De George FV, Engle MA, Passarge E: Possible teratogenicity of trimethadione and paramethadione. Lancet 2:261–262, 1970.
8. Zackai EH, Mellman WJ, Nefderer B, Hanson JW: The fetal trimethadione syndrome. J Pediatr 87:280–284, 1975.

9. Nora JJ, Nora AH, Toews H: Lithium, Ebstein anomaly and other congenital heart defects. Lancet 2:594–595, 1974.
10. Saxen I, Saxen L: Association between maternal intake of diazepam and oral clefts. Lancet 2:498, 1975.
11. Safra MJ, Oakley GP, Jr: Association between cleft lip with or without cleft palate and prenatal exposure to diazepam. Lancet 2:478–480, 1975.
12. Heinonen OP, Slone D, Shapiro S: "Birth Defects and Drugs in Pregnancy." Littleton, Massachusetts: Publishing Sciences Group, Inc., 1977.
13. Shepard TH: "Catalog of Teratogenic Agents," Ed 2. Baltimore: The Johns Hopkins University Press, 1976.
14. Shepard TH: Teratogenicity from drugs – An increasing problem. Disease-a-Month, June 1974.
15. Anonymous: Diagnostic x-rays are no cause for abortion – But caution is advised. JAMA 236:2269; 2277; 2279, 1976.

Drug and Chemical Risks to the Fetus: Occupational Hazards for Medical Personnel

Michael T. Mennuti, MD

Teratogenic risks to medical personnel should be a concern to all of us, not only from a scientific point of view but also for the effects they may have on our families and those of our co-workers. In spite of this, even when compared to other major industries, we have relatively little information or reasonable guidelines to offer hospital personnel. Special risks for those of us in clinical medicine or in medical research may be identified among four categories: drug usage, occupational exposure to drugs or chemicals, viral exposure, and radiation. The first two areas will be the subject of this paper.

VOLUNTARY DRUG USE

Little information is available regarding drug usage by hospital personnel. It seems plausible to consider that this may be increased in physicians primarily on the basis of accessibility. This may also be true for other hospital personnel who have access to medication or who through daily contact with physicians may obtain prescription medication without the benefit of a formal doctor–patient relationship. Statements that narcotic addiction is an occupational hazard of physicians support this presumption [1, 2]. Although a number of other factors have been implicated as predisposing to this problem (eg, fatigue, depression, etc), accessibility is usually the most prominently mentioned. Since this problem may often not be reported or recorded, estimates of its frequency may only represent the "tip of the iceberg." These observations are further supported by the finding of an increased use of mood-altering drugs by physicians. In a prospective 20-year study an increased use of sedatives, tranquilizers, and stimulants was found in 45 physicians when compared to 90 matched controls who were selected as college classmates [3]. Notably, all of the subjects were preselected for "psychological soundness" at the inception of the study. Although this study was conducted in

Drug and Chemical Risks to the Fetus and Newborn: 41–47

men, it is likely that women physicians and other health personnel who might be pregnant may also represent a higher risk group for use of these drugs, about which there is some concern for the exposed fetus.

The admonition that physicians should consider themselves a high-risk group for drug usage should probably be extended to all medical personnel. Especially, we should advise against using drugs that will "make us feel better" simply because such drugs are easily accessible. Although the remainder of this paper will deal with occupational exposure, it is quite possible that voluntary drug use may be the more important teratogenic risk for medical personnel and certainly one that might be more easily prevented.

OCCUPATIONAL EXPOSURES

In the recent past there has been a great deal of concern regarding two frequent exposures for a number of medical personnel and the possible association of these with infertility, abortion, or congenital malformation. These are exposure to volatile anesthetics and to hexachlorophene.

Anesthetics

It is reasonable that concerns arose regarding volatile anesthetics because of their known effects on cellular division and respiration [4]. A number of studies have demonstrated teratogenicity in several species [5]. Both the qualitative and quantitative abnormalities observed have led to the suggestion that the teratogenic effect might possibly be charcteristic of anesthetic agents in general rather than specific for a particular agent. In this regard, it has also been postulated that the efects observed may be the results of hypoxia with deep anesthesia rather than agent-specific.

Nevertheless, since anesthetic gases are found in varying concentrations in operating rooms and in the expired air from personnel, the effects of chronic exposure to rather low levels in humans must be considered [6]. The possibility that this exposure might lead to an increased abortion rate was first reported in the Russian literature [7]. This was followed by a report from Denmark of a similar finding [8]. The latter study suffers from the flaw of comparing the subjects' reproductive outcome at younger ages with data obtained later in life. More recent surveys have controlled for such factors as age and smoking history. Most of these studies have been conducted by the retrospective questionnaire method. Two groups have reported their findings in three large surveys of exposed personnel.

In an early study, Knill-Jones et al compared reproductive performance in 563 married women anesthetists and 828 control women physicians [9]. As a group anesthetists did not differ significantly from controls with respect to frequency of abortion. Anesthetists at work however had a significantly higher risk of abortion (18.2%) than the control group (14.7%) but did not differ significantly from anesthetists not at work. In contrast the frequency of malformations was significantly higher in children born to anesthetists who worked (6.5%) than in those not at work (2.5%) but did not differ significantly from controls (4.9%). Unexplained infertility occurred in 12% of anesthetists compared to 6% of controls. In a later study by the same authors, male and female physicians in the United Kingdom were surveyed [10]. There was no difference observed in abortion rate, infertility, or major congenital anomalies related to paternal exposure. Once again maternal exposure was associated with a higher abortion rate (15.5%) than in nonexposed couples (10.9%). No difference in frequency of major congenital anomalies was observed with maternal exposure.

Several similar studies have been conducted in the United States, which also indicate a higher frequency of miscarriage in exposed women. In an interview study that compared operating room nurses to general duty nurses and female anesthetists to other physicians, both exposed groups had a substantially higher frequency of spontaneous abortions (29.7% and 37.8%) when compared to the controls (8.8% and 10.3%) [11]. It was noted in this study that spontaneous abortions ocurred earlier in the pregnancies of exposed women than in controls (eighth vs tenth week of gestation). The authors felt that this observation further suggested a fetal lethality, possibly due to the anesthetic gases. One might, however, as easily conclude that these observations indicate a more frequent recognition of early abortion by operating room personnel.

The results of a large collaborative questionnaire study in the United States compared members of six national societies [12]. Interestingly, rates of spontaneous abortion were higher in women members of two of the three societies with potential exposure but not significantly different for the third when compared to unexposed controls. Additionally within the three at-risk societies, exposed members had a significantly higher rate of abortion than unexposed members in only one group. These findings are somewhat divergent from those observed in the earlier British study. That there appeared to be no increase in the frequency of abortion in wives of exposed males is in agreement with the results of the later British survey. The frequency of malformation in children of both exposed female and male respondents was increased. Although no specific malformation pattern emerged, the excess could be accounted for by some of the most common multifactorial defects. Despite inconsistencies between the various subgroups within these studies and between the individual studies, when the results of these three large surveys were combined, in addition to the higher frequency of abortion in exposed females, an increased frequency of congenital abnormalities was observed in offspring of both exposed male and female respondents [13].

Because concentrations of anesthetic gases during dental surgery are several times higher than those found in general operating rooms, a survey of reproductive performance of wives of dentists would be expected to be more indicative of the effects of paternal exposure. Interestingly, the abortion rate for wives of exposed dentists (16.0%) was significantly higher than for wives of unexposed dentists (9.0%) [14]. In contrast to the observations of the combined retrospective surveys, congenital abnormalities wre not significantly increased when there had been this higher level paternal exposure.

Two authors have critically reviewed the findings of many of these studies and have concluded that a cause–effect relationship between chronic exposure to trace levels of anesthetic gases and reproductive failure has not been established [4, 5]. In addition to the usual pitfalls often encountered in the design of retrospective questionnaires, spontaneous abortion data may be particularly fraught with error. The incidence of early spontaneous abortion is quite high, variable, and not substantially different from the rates reported in these studies. As previously mentioned, correction for maternal age is critically important based on the association of an age-related incidence of chromosome abnormalities that may account for a substantial proportion of spontaneous abortions. In addition, previous history of spontaneous or induced abortion may influence the likelihood of subsequent abortion independent of exposure. The results of retrospective questionnaires of the type reviewed may be influenced by frequency of diagnosis in certain groups of individuals or perhaps more importantly by unconfirmed self-diagnosis. When comparing professional women at work to their peers not at work, it seems likely that the group of women who continue to work may be included with those who have reproductive failure, while those who no longer work are more likely to have normal reproductive histories. Environmental factors other than anesthetic gases may account for the findings in these studies. For example, it has been suggested that the "stress" of the operating room may be an important consideration and that perhaps intensive care nurses would serve as better "controls" for operating room nurses than general duty nurses.

The actual reproductive risk associated with this exposure continues to be a cause for concern and debate [15–18]. Since a higher risk of abortion in pregnancies of exposed women is the most consistent finding of these studies, it would seem that prospective monitoring of the abortuses in these cases would be a useful approach to elucidating this risk. With the development of new cytogenetic techniques and a decreased occurrence of criminally induced abortion, an even higher frequency of chromosome abnormalities in first trimester abortuses has been observed than was in the past. With this background information and correlation with the morphologic findings in abortuses, several authors have proposed that surveillance of spontaneous abortions should be an increasingly powerful tool for environmental monitoring [19, 20].

The possibility that chronic exposure to trace concentrations of anesthetic gases *may* have a causal association with reproductive failure raises questions regarding reducing or eliminating this possible risk. As with other environmental agents that may have a teratogenic risk, it is not known whether there is an important "threshold" level of exposure. At present, the most reasonable recommendation is to reduce the exposure to the lowest possible limit consistent with cost.

A reduction in anesthetic contamination in the operating room may be achieved by the removal of excess circuit gases (scavenging), elimination of equipment leakage, and avoiding techniques that allow spill of volatile agents. These approaches have been reviewed in detail by Lecky [21]. Personnel working in operating rooms should be made aware of these issues in order to enlist their cooperation in reducing anesthetic contamination and also to help them decide whether they wish to continue working in the operating room area during pregnancy. It seems reasonable that women, especially those with a history of previous pregnancy loss, may request assignment to rooms with scavenging equipment or perhaps other areas of their department during early pregnancy.

Hexachlorophene

Following the demonstration of absorption and neurotoxicity of hexachlorophene (HCP) in newborns, it was not unexpected that concerns would arise regarding teratogenicity.

Doctor Hildegard Halling, a Swedish physician at a chronic disease hospital, called attention to this after observing a "cluster" of infants with somewhat similar malformations born to women employees who washed frequently with HCP-containing detergent [22, 23]. By adding these cases to several other "clusters" observed in similar institutions and comparing the frequency of malformations to that in children of unexposed women, it was concluded that there was a teratogenic risk related to this exposure. It has been argued, however, that inclusion of the initial exposed cases, which were selected on the basis of malformation rather than on the basis of exposure, has biased these observations [24]. Additionally, the frequency of serious malformation in the control group was lower than expected for the general population. These findings prompted a subsequent investigation of obstetrical outcome in hospital personnel by the National Board of Health and Welfare in Sweden. In this study perinatal death rates and malformation in children of these workers were surveyed for 1973–1975. No significant difference was found except for an excess of perinatal deaths in the hospital workers offspring in 1973 only. Neither the frequency of perinatal death nor malformation differed between 3,007 infants born to women who worked in hospitals in which HCP was used frequently when compared to 1,653 infants born to women who worked in hospitals in which HCP was not used or was used infrequently [25]. Thus the nature and level of this potential risk are unclear. Until further information is available it would seem that if exposure is minimized there would appear to be no cause for undue concern.

CONCLUSION

It is important that we continue to be alert for other teratogenic risks to medical personnel. It is also apparent that there is a need for considerably more information regarding the exposures discussed in this paper. This is true not only for the potential prevention of reproductive wastage or birth defects but also to avoid undue anxiety or elective abortion following exposure during pregnancy. Of the factors that lead to counseling and possibly to termination of pregnancy following drug or chemical exposure, a heightened awareness of birth defects and their burden is especially prevalent among medical personnel. Counseling and decision making in this circumstance is also more difficult when the patient has access to animal studies, case reports, opinion papers, and perhaps well-intentioned "unofficial consultations." Although the actual risks associated with the agents that have been discussed may be questioned, until further information is available, it seems prudent to minimize exposure when possible. This is advisable if only to reduce anxiety or the possibility of a decision for abortion based on an ill-defined risk.

REFERENCES

1. Green RC, Carroll GJ, Buxton WD, Drug addiction among physicians: The Virginia experience. JAMA 236:1372, 1976.
2. Anslinger HJ: Interview. Mod Med 25:170–191, 1957.
3. Vaillant GE, Brighton JR, McArthur C: Physicians' use of mood-altering drugs: A 20-year follow-up report. N Engl J Med 282:365–370, 1970.
4. Smith BE: Teratology in anesthesia. Clin Obstet Gynecol 17:145–148, 1974.
5. Ferstandig LL: Trace concentrations of anesthetic gases: A critical review of their disease potential. Anesth Analg 57:328–345, 1978.
6. Whitcher CE, Cohen EN, Trudell JR: Chronic exposure to anesthetic gases in the operating room. Anesthesiology 35:348–353, 1974.
7. Vaisman AL: Working conditions in surgery and their effect on the health of anesthesiologists. Eksp Khir Anesteziol 3:44–48, 1967.
8. Askrog V, Harvald B: Teratogenic effects of inhalation anesthetics. Nord Med 83:498–500, 1970.
9. Knill-Jones RP, Moir DD, Rodriques LV, Spence AA: Anaesthetic practice and pregnancy: Controlled survey of women anaesthetists in the United Kingdom. Lancet 1: 1326–1328, 1972.
10. Knill-Jones RP, Newman BJ, Spence AA: Anaesthetic practice and pregnancy: Controlled survey of male anaesthetists in the United Kingdom. Lancet 2:807–809, 1975.
11. Cohen EN, Bellville JW, Brown BW: Anesthesia, pregnancy, and miscarriage: A study of oerating room nurses and anesthetists. Anesthesiology 35:343–347, 1971.
12. Cohen EN, Brown BW, Bruse DL, et al: Occupational disease among operating room personnel: A national study. Anesthesiology 41:321–340, 1974.
13. Spence AA, et al: Occupational hazards for operating room-based physicians: Analysis of data from the United States and the United Kingdom. JAMA 238:955–959, 1977.
14. Cohen EN, Brown BW, Bruce DL, et al: A survey of anesthetic health hazards among dentists. JAm Dent Assoc 90:1291–1296, 1975.

15. Ruston DI: Anaesthetics and abortions: Lancet 2.141, 1976.
16. Tomlin PJ: Teratogenic effects of waste anaesthetic gases. Br Med J Jan: 108, 1978.
17. Tomlin PJ: Teratogenic effects of waste anaesthetic gases. Br Med J Feb: 300, 1978.
18. McPherson K, Smith P, Vessey M: Teratogenic effects of waste anaesthetic gases. Br Med J Feb:437–438, 1978.
19. Oakley GP Jr: The use of human abortuses in the search for teratogens. In U.S. Dept HEW: "Methods for Detection of Environmental Agents that Produce Congenital Defects, 1975." Washington, DC: US Government Printing Office, 1975, p 189–196.
20. Kline J, et al: Surveillance of spontaneous abortions: Power in environmental monitoring. Am J Epidemiol 106:345–350, 1977.
21. Lecky JH: The mechanical aspects of anesthetic pollution control. Anesth Analog 56: 769–776, 1977.
22. Halling H: Suspected link between exposure to hexachlorophene and birth of malformed infants. Lakartidningen 74:542–546, 1977.
23. Check W: New study shows hexachlorophene is teratogenic in humans. JAMA 240:513–514, 1978.
24. Kallen B: Hexachlorophene teratogenicity in humans disputed. JAMA 240:1585–1586, 1978.
25. Baltzar B, Ericson A, Kallen B: Pregnancy outcome among women working in Swedish hospitals. N Engl J Med 300:627–628, 1979.

Male Mediated Drug Effects on Offspring

Lester F. Soyka, MD, and Justin M. Joffe, PhD

The goal of this chapter is to introduce a new concept, namely that drug and chemical exposure of a male can affect his progeny. It is generally accepted that drugs administered to pregnant animals or humans may have untoward effects on the fetus and newborn. While maternally mediated teratogenesis is a well established phenomenon in reproductive biology, its clinical significance was not widely recognized and accepted until the thalidomide catastrophe. Thalidomide remains a unique drug in that it is noncytotoxic but has a selective, devastating effect on the fetus as even a few doses, administered at a precise critical period, produce severe limb deformities. However, the tragedy of these deformed children brought about widespread recognition of the wide variety of effects of drugs administered to pregnant women. While the fields of investigation of drug passage across the placenta, critical stages of development, and so forth, are still in their infancy, this paper will be concerned with a field on the verge of birth, and perhaps a premature birth at that. Based on our work and on a literature survey, we propose that chemical agents can act through the sire to exhibit adverse effects on the outcome of pregnancy.

All of the chemical agents suspected of having adverse effects on progeny when administered to males are known to exert deleterious effects on the fetus and newborn when administered to pregnant females. In at least one study, adverse effects were more pronounced when both parents were drug treated. However, for the sake of clarity, this paper is limited to those studies in which only the male parent was treated. It bears emphasizing that in all the studies described here the female is "drug-naive."

EXPERIMENTAL STUDIES

Our studies arose from a serendipitous observation made by the late Dr. Durwood J. Smith, together with Dr. Justin Joffe, during studies of drugs administered to pregnant rats. As a control in one experiment, morphine was administered to male rats; this resulted in extremely high neonatal mortality and

Drug and Chemical Risks to the Fetus and Newborn: 49–66

prompted these investigators to repeat the study under controlled conditions [1]. The neonatal survival of 166 live offspring sired by male rats treated with morphine sulfate and that of 145 live offspring sired by male rats treated with methadone was remarkably decreased compared to controls (Fig. 1). Only 66% of the offspring sired by morphine-treated males and only 26% of those sired by methadone-treated males survived to 21 days of age.

Variability among the outcome of individual litters proved to be a general phenomenon seen in all of our experiments over the past three years. For example, Figure 2 presents data on individual litter outcome of controls, a low-dose methadone group, and a high-dose methadone group [1]. The drug was put in the drinking water for 24 hours prior to mating. Four impregnated females in each of the drug-treated groups did not deliver live offspring, versus only two in the control group. The excessive mortality was seen in virtually all litters but was more pronounced in the high-dose methadone group. Nevertheless, one small litter had no deaths, whereas one litter had no survivors.

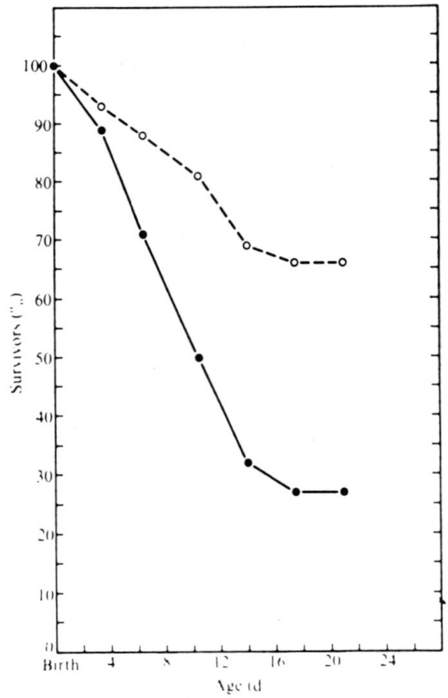

Fig. 1. Neonatal (birth–21 days of age) survival of 166 offspring sired by male rats pretreated with morphine sulfate (open circles) and 145 offspring sired by male rats pretreated with methadone hydrochloride (closed circles). Offspring of untreated males had survival rates of 90–95%. From Nature 253:202–203, 1975 [1].

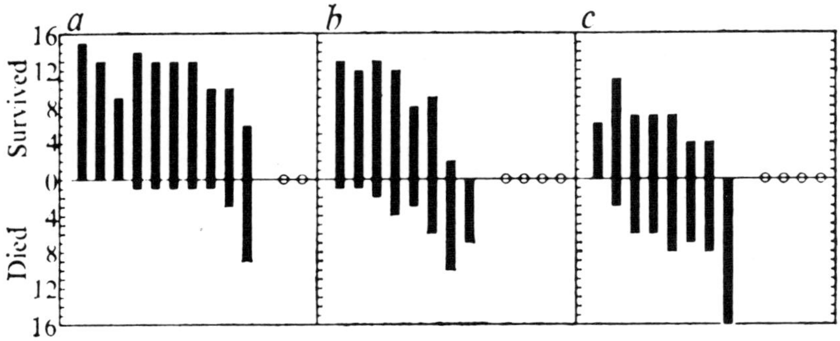

Fig. 2. Survival and deaths in each litter sired by a) control, b) low-dose, and c) high-dose methadone-treated male rats. Open circles indicate impregnated females that did not deliver offspring. From Nature 253:202–203, 1975 [1].

Other prominent effects of paternal methadone were decreased birthweights and weaning weights and an increase in the number of small litters [2,3]. These effects were found in studies following the general design shown in Figure 3. Methadone, 10 mg/kg, was administered subcutaneously at 1000 hours. Duration of treatment varied from one to 12 days in various studies. Males were caged overnight with drug-naive females. Females were examined for the presence of sperm, and those with positive vaginal smears were isolated to await delivery. At the time of delivery, pups were counted, sexed, and weighed, and in some studies, tattooed to allow follow-up of individual outcome. Pups were counted at two-day intervals thereafter until weaning at 21 days of age, when they were again weighed. In some studies behavioral testing in the open field was carried out, as well as weighing and evaluation of reproductive performance.

The drug-induced lowering of birthweight was confounded by an effect of prior copulation on birthweights. Copulation within a few days of the test mating resulted in increased birthweights of litters sired by control males injected with sterile water (Fig. 4). Male and female pups from litters sired by males receiving methadone were significantly lighter at birth than control pups only when the litters were sired by males that had previously copulated. These results suggested that methadone may be acting at a critical time during maturation of spermatozoa. Methadone treatment also affected litter size (Fig. 5). There were more litters born with an abnormally low number of pups (two to six per litter) in the methadone-sired group. This difference was statistically significant, with a Fisher exact probability of 0.02.

The neonatal mortality data from five experiments, totaling 2,611 methadone offspring compared to 1,565 control pups, are summarized in Figure 6. Although excessive mortality was found in every study, the absolute rates varied from 4% to 74%, depending on dose, duration of treatment, etc. In each experiment the

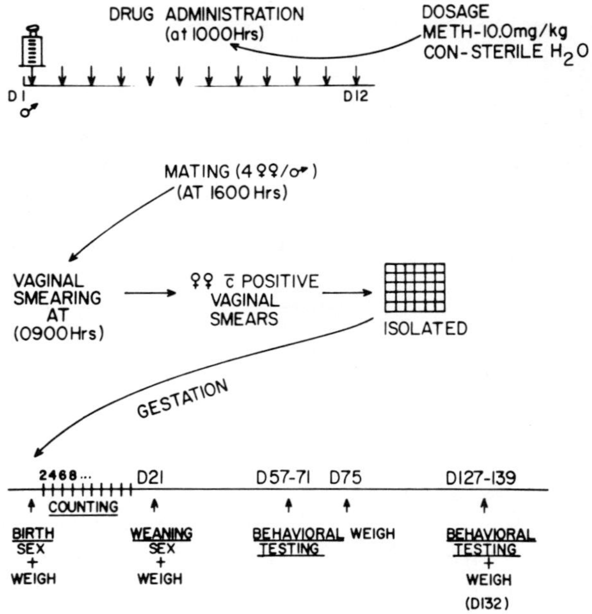

Fig. 3. Protocol for studies of methadone treatment of male rats on their progeny.

mortality of the methadone-sired offspring was twice that of concurrent control litters, and in one instance it was very much higher. Summing over experiments, the neonatal mortality of methadone-sired pups averaged 25% as compared to 8% of controls.

In all studies deaths occurred chiefly between eight and 14 days of age (Fig. 7). In this particular study, the rate was higher among males; this was a general trend but not invariable. Examined in another fashion (Fig. 8), plotting deaths/100 survivors against postnatal age, a peak of deaths was noted in the first two days of life in the methadone progeny, with a second and larger peak at the tenth to twelfth postnatal day. This was also the peak time for deaths among the control offspring, suggesting an accentuation of a fundamental biologic phenomenon. Alternatively, one can speculate that this peak of deaths in control offspring was also somehow related to chemical exposure.

Chronic administration of methadone, that is for 20–30 days prior to the test mating, resulted in litters of normal size, birthweight, and neonatal viatility [4]. In addition, mating after three months of daily methadone revealed no differences from controls in number of ova failing to implant, early or late fetal deaths, or corpora lutea count in the dominant lethal test of Epstein and Röhrborn [5].

Since narcotic analgesics are known to reduce serum luteinizing hormone and serum testosterone concentrations, in a later study we administered testosterone concurrently with methadone [6]. The neonatal survival was significantly improved compared to litters of methadone-treated males; methadone, 42/142 vs methadone plus testosterone, 22/159 (χ^2 = 11.10, P < 0.001). Because we lack "testosterone-only" and "vehicle-only" controls for these studies, we are not able to say at this time that testosterone completely normalized outcome.

Administration of testosterone concurrently with methadone resulted in increased seminal vesicle weight; prostate weight was also increased, though the increase was not statistically significant. These findings indicate that the conversion of testosterone to its active 5-alpha-dihydro metabolite was not blocked in these target tissues. One can only speculate whether these changes – that is, maintenance of normal seminal vesicle and prostate weights – relate causally to the improved neonatal survival.

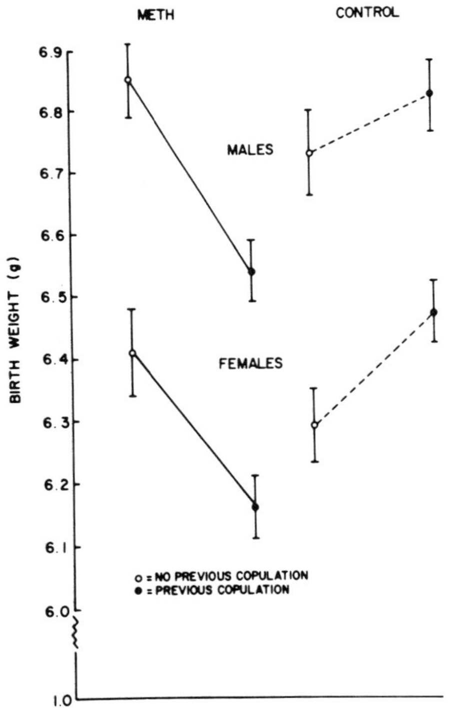

Fig. 4. Effect of methadone treatment (METH) and of prior copulation on birthweights of male and female rats. Values are mean ± SEM. From Toxicol Appl Pharmacol 45:797, 1978 [3].

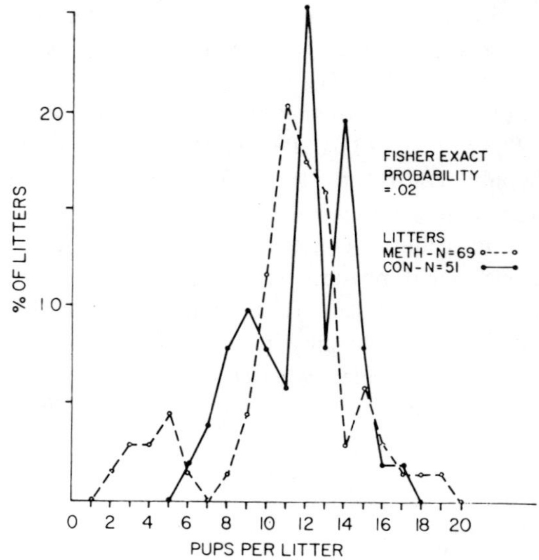

Fig. 5. Effect of methadone treatment of male rats on number of pups per litter. The number of small-sized litters (2–6 pups/litter) was significantly increased among the 69 methadone (METH)-sired litters vs the 51 control (CON) litters ($P < 0.02$, Fisher exact probability).

Additional studies were based on an abbreviated design in which drugs were administered once or twice daily for three or four days, followed by overnight mating with a proestrous drug-naive virgin female, and observations were made of birthweight, sex and number, neonatal mortality, and weaning weight.

Caffeine, 50 mg/kg/day for four days, resulted in significantly increased neonatal mortality (Fig. 9). Moreover, three drug-treated males failed to mate, and five females with a positive vaginal smear for sperm failed to deliver. As with methadone, the effect on neonatal survival was extreme in some litters: three small litters had no survivors, whereas two normal-sized litters had no deaths. One-tenth the dose of caffeine (5 mg/kg/day for four days) resulted in a neonatal mortality rate of approximately 20%, roughly double that of the controls, but clearly less than the 37% mortality found after 50 mg/kg/day. The time course of deaths was similar to that seen among the methadone-sired pups, with most deaths occurring from eight to 14 days of age (Fig. 10).

Our data with propoxyphene, a nonaddictive narcotic analgesic that is chemically related to methadone and marketed as Darvon, were inconclusive because of lack of a dose-response relationship (Fig. 11). Two dose schedules were studied. Schedule A was 30, 40, and then 80 mg/kg subcutaneously at 0900 hours on three successive days and resulted in a neonatal mortality rate of 36%. Deaths occurred in all litters save the smallest. Dose schedule B, 40, 80, and 120 mg/kg, resulted in litters that were less affected, although one impregnated female failed

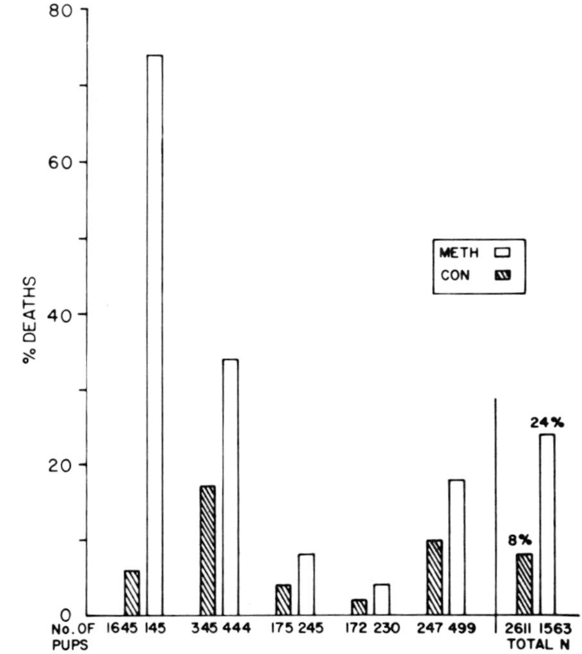

Fig. 6. Neonatal mortality rates from five experiments conducted over a three-year period. Methadone treatment was of male rats only, and varied in regard to dose, duration, and route of administration. The bars on the right summarize the data.

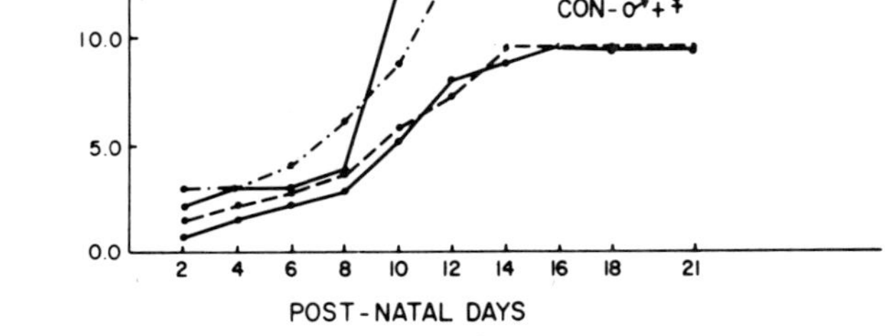

Fig. 7. Time course of deaths of offspring of methadone-treated male rats. Days indicate postnatal age.

to deliver. No small litters were found, and the neonatal mortality rate was 11%, not significantly different from controls in this experiment. It should be noted that this was a high rate for our controls, and therefore the figure of 11% for the propoxyphene progeny may be a significant drug effect. This lack of an apparent dose response with propoxyphene and our limited data with caffeine lead us to consider these data as preliminary.

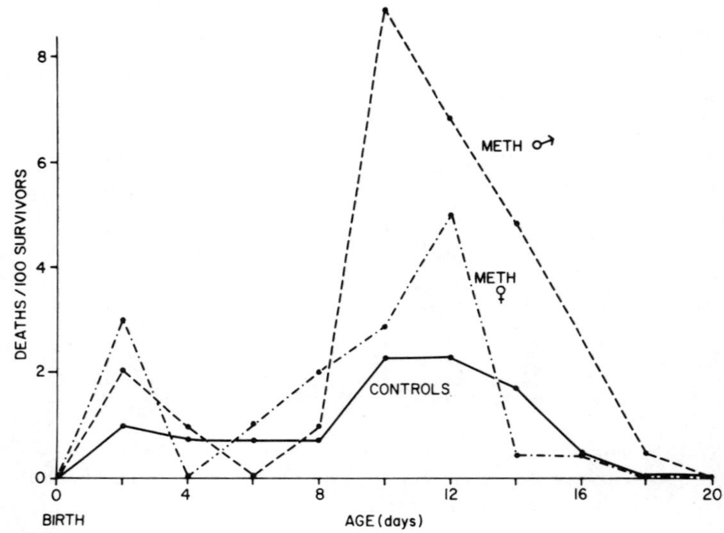

Fig. 8. Incidence of deaths/100 survivors of offspring of methadone-treated male rats.

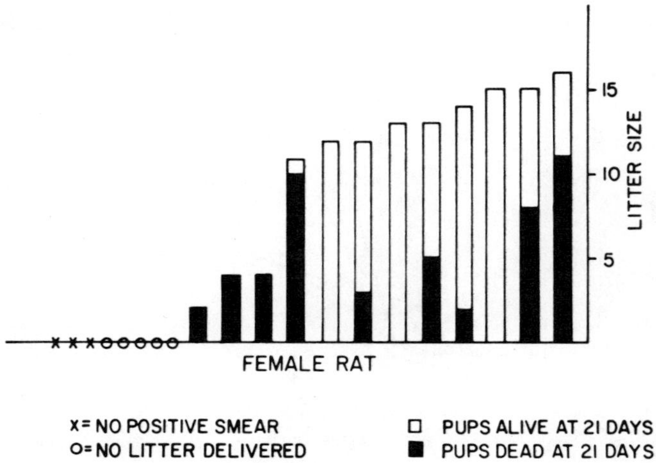

Fig. 9. Litter size and neonatal deaths/litter of offspring sired by male rats treated with caffeine, 25 mg/kg subcutaneously twice daily for four days, prior to mating.

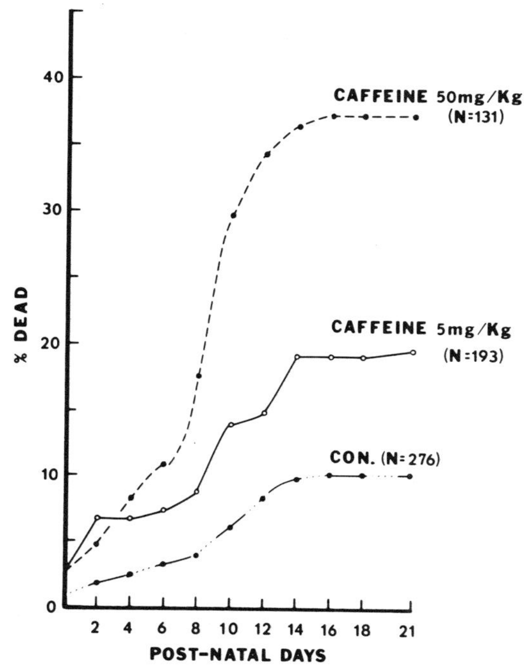

Fig. 10. Time course and cumulative neonatal mortality rates for offspring of males treated with caffeine, 50 mg/kg/day subcutaneously for four days, caffeine, 5 mg/kg/day subcutaneously for four days, or sterile water (CON).

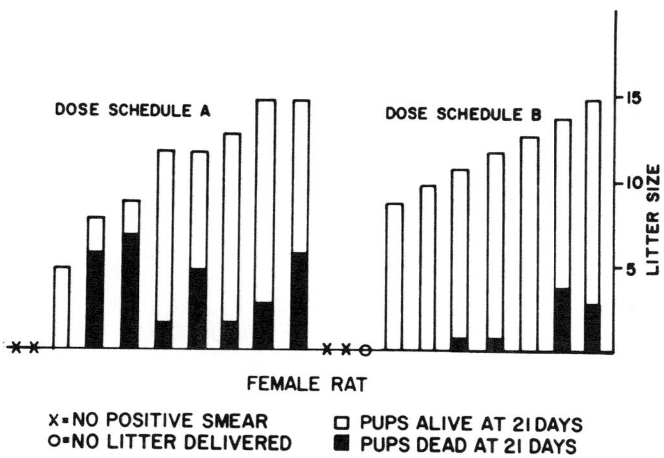

Fig. 11. Litter size and neonatal deaths/litter of offspring sired by male rats treated with propoxyphene. Dose schedule A was 30, 40, and 80 mg/kg subcutaneously at 0900 hours on each of three successive days; dose schedule B was 40, 80, and 120 mg/kg. The neonatal mortality rate of the 89 offspring of group A was 35%, and for the 84 group B offspring it was 117.

In addition to our findings, adverse effects on progeny of five species have been reported for lead, morphine, thalidomide, caffeine, and ethanol (Table I). Details of these findings are contained in our recent literature review [7]. Despite variations in species, agents, dosage, timing of administration, and a variety of other parameters, three effects emerge consistently: decreased litter sizes, lower birthweights (intrauterine growth retardation), and increased neonatal mortality.

CLINICAL STUDIES

Clinical data are scant and difficult to interpret (Table II). Many methodological problems prevent the demonstration of an unequivocal relationship between paternal drug ingestion and perinatal outcome. Authors of some very old

TABLE I. Summary of Adverse Effects of Drugs and Chemicals Administered to Male Mammals Prior to Mating on Their Progeny*

Species	Effects	Reference	Year
Lead			
Rabbit	Decreased litter size, birthweight, survival	[8]	1914
Guinea pig	Decreased birthweight, survival, weight gain	[9]	1915
Rat	Decreased litter size, birthweight, survival	[10]	1971
Rat	Decreased learning ability – T-maze	[11]	1975
Morphine			
Mouse	Decreased weight – F_1 + F_2 generations	[12]	1974
Ethanol			
Guinea pig	Intrauterine deaths, decreased postnatal survival (F_1 – F_3 generations)	[13]	1913
Mouse	No significant effects on sex ratio, prenatal mortality	[14a,b] [14c]	1926 1927
Guinea pig	No significant effects on birthweight, sex ratio, pre/postnatal mortality	[15]	1932
Mouse	Intrauterine deaths	[16]	1975
Rat	Decreased litter size and fetal size	[17]	1976
Caffeine			
Hamster	Skewing of sex ratio toward females	[18]	1975
Thalidomide			
Rabbit	Decreased birthweight, litter size, survival, increased malformations	[19]	1964

*Additional information is available on effects of lead [8], alcohol, and ether [20] on chickens. Deleterious effects of caffeine treatment have been reported on the testes of roosters and their fertility [21]. Effects of combined maternal and paternal ingestion of lead in rats have also been reported [22,23].

TABLE II. Summary of Adverse Effects of Drug Exposure on the Reproductive Performance of Men

Agent	Effects	Reference	Year
Lead	Increased spontaneous abortions, neonatal mortality	[24]	1860
	Reduced family size	[25]	1908
	Increased spontaneous abortions	[26]	1910
	Increased spontaneous abortions, stillbirths, neonatal mortality	[27]	1911
Anesthetic gases	Increased spontaneous abortions, congenital anomalies	[28]	1974
	Increased spontaneous abortions	[29]	1975
Cigarettes	Increased incidence of low-birthweight (LBW) infants, increased neonatal mortality, and congenital anomalies in LBW infants	[30]	1971
Caffeine	Increased reproductive loss (spontaneous abortions, stillbirths, premature births)	[31]	1977

papers, dating back to 1860, were concerned with the reproductive performance of men involved in trades in which there was excessive exposure to lead. The severity and duration of this exposure is far beyond that which would be tolerated as an occupational hazard today. Effects such as increased rates of spontaneous abortions, stillbirths, neonatal mortality, and reduced family size were found in four reports [24–27]. Perhaps more relevant are the results of nationwide surveys of operating room personnel and of dentists and oral surgeons. An increased number, but not to a level of statistical significance, of spontaneous abortions and congenital anomalies was found among offspring of male dentists and anesthetists exposed to volatile anesthetics [28,29].

The extensive studies of Yerushalmy [30] on influences on pregnancy outcome detected an increased incidence of low-birthweight infants as well as increased neonatal mortality and congenital anomalies in low-birthweight infants whose fathers were cigarette smokers. We were surprised that we were unable to find additional studies that would confirm or deny this important observation.

In a study of residents of Salt Lake City, where it was felt that drug, alcohol, and caffeine ingestion would be very low, an increase in spontaneous abortions, stillbirths, and premature births among offspring sired by fathers who drank coffee and other caffeine-containing beverages and whose mothers did not was reported [31]. However, the very high incidence of these events in this study and the difficulty of controlling for other variables leaves this as a tantalizing but inconclusive observation.

In summary, although the exposure to the substances investigated was generally chronic, the reported effects in humans are similar to those found after acute dosing in animal studies. No controls are reported in the case of lead exposure (the increases are relative to population statistics), and in the cases of anesthetic gases, cigarettes, and caffeine, it is probable that the fathers also differed in their ingestion of other substances. For example, Yerushalmy [30] found that smokers and nonsmokers differed in a number of ways, including consumption of coffee and alcohol. Difficulties such as these make it difficult to pinpoint single drug causal relationships. Nevertheless, the outcomes reported are similar to those found in controlled animal experiments.

FACTORS INFLUENCING MALE-MEDIATED EFFECTS

Only in the case of methadone are data sufficient to deduce factors influencing the nature and severity of the adverse effects on offspring. Those identified include: 1) dose, 2) time of administration in relation to time of mating, 3) duration of administration, and 4) sexual activity during the period of drug administration.

Dose

Increased neonatal mortality was dose-related in our initial studies [1,2]. Variability in individual males' ingestion via self-regulated oral administration precluded definition of a precise dose-response relationship. Using subcutaneous injections to standardize dosage, studies indicated mortality to be significantly higher than that of concurrent controls at a dose of 10 mg/kg/day [3], but not with 5 mg/kg (unpublished data). Doses of 15 or 20 mg/kg/day blocked male sexual activity, precluding definition of a more complete dose-response curve.

Time of Administration Relative to Time of Mating

Death rates in progeny of males ingesting methadone 24–48 hours before mating were lower than the rate when males were dosed during the 24 hours immediately prior to mating [1].

Duration of Administration

The duration of drug exposure was a complex variable. A single dose increased mortality from 3% to 8% [2]. The effect of several days of drug treatment was difficult to define precisely, since tolerance appeared to develop with subacute and chronic treatment [3]. In this respect, it should be noted that the dose was held constant throughout the experiment, whereas the period of sedation following administration of methadone decreased throughout the period of study, indicating central nervous system tolerance.

Sexual Activity During Drug Administration

The cause(s) of intrauterine deaths, as suggested by decreased litter size (Fig. 5), and of neonatal mortality (Fig. 6), are largely unknown. Badr and Badr [16] proposed a dominant lethal mutation to explain in utero deaths of offspring sired by ethanol-treated mice. We have attempted to relate risk of death to body weight at birth (32). Deaths occurred more frequently in pups with birthweights lower than average when sired by methadone-treated or propoxyphene-treated male rats, but in the heavier pups in the case of caffeine. Examination of the offspring in our studies has failed to reveal gross congenital anomalies. Whatever cause is postulated must be compatible with our consistent observation of a peak incidence of deaths occurring eight to 14 days after birth (Figs. 7 and 8).

MECHANISMS OF DRUG ACTION

Stowe and Goyer [10] found the RNA content of rat testes was significantly lowered by dietary administration of lead, and they concluded that ribosomal activity and protein synthesis were impaired. In studies of ethanol ingestion by male mice, determination of either litter size or uterine contents indicated early fetal demise without an effect on fertility, leading to a postulate of lethal mutation [16]. Such a mechanism could account for the finding of an increased number of small litters in the methadone studies. We were unable to demonstrate a dominant lethal effect by the technique of Epstein and Röhrborn [5] after chronic methadone administration, but neither was there an increase in neonatal mortality with this protocol [4]. We found no evidence for a genetic defect in producing an F_2 generation by mating of offspring of methadone-treated males [3]. Falek et al [33] conducted a careful cytogenic study of leukocytes from 16 multiple drug users who were receiving methadone. They observed 2.56% chromatid and isochromatid breaks, exchange figures, and dicentric chromosomes in multiple drug users versus 0.39% in the control population. They then conducted an in vitro study to evaluate the effects of varying concentrations of methadone, morphine, and quinine on leukocytes from cord blood. Doses varying from 1/12 to three times the therapeutic concentration were introduced at 24, 48, and 68 hours into 72-hour leukocyte cultures without producing an increase in chromosome damage. Friedler and Wurster-Hill [34] found no consistent abnormalities in the chromosomes cultured from 17 control and 18 offspring of morphine-treated males and drug-naive females.

Drugs and/or Metabolite(s) in Seminal Fluid

Lutwak-Mann et al [35] found thalidomide and its metabolites in appreciable quantities in the semen of rabbits after oral administration. After subcutaneous administration of ^{14}C-methadone to male rats, radioactivity was present in the copulation plugs of females (unpublished observation). Gerber and Lynn [36] found methadone in the semen of seven clients of a methadone maintenance clinic, with concentration ratios of 0.8–4.7 relative to serum. Swanson et al [37] found phenytoin in the semen of rabbits and man in concentrations of 0.2 relative to plasma.

Whereas the mere presence of a chemical in semen does not prove that it is pharmacologically active, there exist a number of possible ways in which the offspring might be affected. First, a variety of chemicals have been shown to reduce or abolish motility of human sperm in vitro [38]. More relevant perhaps, impaired sperm motility has been found in man following anticonvulsant therapy [39] and in heroin users and clients of a methadone maintenance program [40]. Reduced motility, possibly coupled with impaired viability, might account for impaired fertility and decreased litter size.

Second, drugs in the semen might have an influence on the uterus, either locally or indirectly, following systemic absorption. Either could result in effects on the location and distribution of implantation sites, placentation, etc. Such a mechanism is suggested by findings that estrogens transported in semen to the female rat during mating affect fertility; females mated to male rats receiving estrogen showed hypertrophy and hyperplasia of uterine tissue, accompanied by increased uterine weight on day 1 of pregnancy, as well as alterations in ova transport that resulted in reduced recovery of cleaved ova from day 2 of pregnancy on [41].

The possibility of effects on the fetus due to systemic absorption appears implausible given the very small quantity of drug that would be available intravaginally. However, two lines of evidence make it inappropriate to exclude this possibility from further consideration. Drugs are rapidly absorbed through the vaginal mucosa, as demonstrated in animal experiments [42] and in clinical reports [43]. In addition, one woman developed severe vaginitis following intercourse during the first three to four days after her husband's ingestion of vinblastine [44].

Other Alterations of the Semen

Narcotics produce a variety of effects on the male reproductive system, with morphine found to cause a reduction in the secretory content of seminal vesicles in rats [45] and methadone (but not heroin) ingestion found to be related to a reduction of over 50% in ejaculate volume and seminal vesicle and prostatic secretions in man [40]. In the latter study, sperm motility in heroin and methadone users was found to be substantially lower than that of control males. It is possible that impaired sperm motility or reduced viability might be due to drug-induced alterations in the volume or composition of the seminal fluid rather than to the presence of the drug or its metabolites. Investigation of prostaglandin content would be of interest since prostaglandins have been implicated in sperm transport and fertilization [46]. Such changes might constitute a final common pathway for a variety of agents administered to the male.

Indirect Effects as a Result of a "Changed Male"

Methadone administration produces several changes, including a loss of body weight, an acute fall in serum luteinizing hormone and testosterone levels, and reduced sexual behavior. Although loss of body weight may play a role in the case of ethanol, where weight loss has sometimes been substantial [17], it does not seem responsible for the effects on progeny we have found, since deleterious effects on perinatal survival and birthweight were most pronounced in matings during the first four days of methadone administration, a time when weight loss was minimal [3]. In addition, effects on the progeny were detected in other studies where methadone was administered for only one or two days [1,2].

Cicero et al [45, 47–51] found that body weight and food and water intake of rats did not change during the three days following implantation of a morphine pellet, whereas during this time prostate and seminal vesicle weight decreased significantly, and there was an 87% fall in serum testosterone concentrations. We found that seminal vesicle weights but not testes weights were significantly decreased by methadone treatment [4]. This is similar to the effect reported by Cicero et al and may be due to decreased testosterone levels. Cicero et al found that by one or two hours after administration of morphine, serum luteinizing hormone levels fell, followed by decreased serum testosterone levels, and decreased prostate and seminal vesicle weights and secretion volume. These effects of narcotics were stereospecific, being more pronounced with the levo-isomer; were blocked by naloxone, a specific narcotic antagonist; and tolerance developed so that serum levels returned to normal after 20 days of chronic morphine administration. Similar effects were found with methadone. However, their conclusion that the adverse effects of narcotics on secondary sex organs were due solely to the decreased serum levels of testosterone caused by the drugs [51] is not entirely consistent with the time course of changes in accessory sexual organs following castration.

Decreased serum testosterone and seminal fluid volume also have been reported in methadone clients. Cushman [52] found that patients receiving 40 mg of methadone or less had significantly higher mean testosterone levels than those receiving more than 40 mg of methadone daily. Mendelson et al [53] reported that patients receiving 80–150 mg of methadone per day showed a significant suppression of plasma testosterone levels, whereas patients maintained on 10–60 mg of methadone had plasma testosterone levels similar to those of controls. Administration of a methadone analog, acetyl methadol, also resulted in decreased testosterone levels [54]. Serum testosterone levels were approximately 43% lower in methadone clients (but not in heroin addicts) than in controls [40]. The suppression of plasma testosterone with large doses of methadone may play a role in the decreased sexual performance of males, though a direct action on brain centers involved in sexual behavior is a reasonable alternative explanation. In our studies of rats, multiple matings particularly were affected, as were the total number of matings [2, 3]. Clinical studies have shown decreased sexual drive and performance in male narcotic addicts. For example, Kreek [55] reported that in interviews with 92 patients who had been in a methadone maintenance program for over three years, 22% complained of decreased libido, and 14% reported decreased orgasm.

In rats, which do not have a functional luteal phase, repeated intromissions prior to ejaculation trigger the tonic secretion of progesterone by stimulating the release of pituitary gonadotrophins. Either by a neuroendocrine mechanism, or by some mechanical means, vaginal stimulation also facilitates passage of sperm through the cervix [56–58]. By decreasing male sexual performance, and thus decreasing vaginal stimulation and resultant sperm transport and progesterone levels, methadone may affect the distribution of implantation sites in the uterus with consequent effects on the maternal-placental-fetal exchange of nutrients and other substances. Other alterations in the male's copulatory behavior also might affect implantation. Shortening of the male's normal postejaculatory refractory period, for example, might deleteriously affect implantation, since intromissions shortly after ejaculation have been shown to inhibit pregnancy [58]. The coital behavior of males following ingestion of methadone has not been studied in sufficient detail to evaluate these possibilities.

SUMMARY AND CONCLUSIONS

Since the thalidomide catastrophe it has become widely recognized that a variety of drugs and chemicals administered during pregnancy have adverse effects on the fetus and newborn. Moreover, chemical agents may produce not only observable congenital malformations but also subtle effects on learning and behavior.

Our work is concerned with a new concept – namely, that drug exposure of a male prior to mating may affect his progeny. While the agents studied to date are also known to have adverse effects on progeny when administered to females, it is to be stressed that in our studies the female was untreated. Our studies have focused on methadone, a synthetic narcotic analgesic widely used in the treatment of heroin abuse. Administration to male rats for one to four days prior to mating resulted in decreased birthweights and weaning weights, increased neonatal mortality, and altered behavior as determined in the open-field test. These effects were not seen in matings after chronic administration (21–32 days) of methadone. The excessive neonatal mortality was significantly reduced by concurrent administration of testosterone. In one study neonatal survival was significantly decreased by administration of caffeine, 50 mg/kg per day for four days, but not by 5 mg/kg. Propoxyphene, a nonaddictive analgesic chemically related to methadone, also resulted in decreased neonatal survival in one study, but no such increase was found in a second study employing a larger dose. Thus results with the latter two drugs must be considered preliminary.

The second part of our study consisted of a review of the literature on paternal drug intake in relation to pregnancy outcome. Adverse effects on progeny of five species have been reported for lead, morphine, thalidomide, caffeine, and ethanol, including decreased litter size, birthweight, survival, and learning ability in a T-maze. In humans, lead, anesthetic gases, cigarettes, and caffeine have been associated with a variety of adverse effects on reproductive performance and outcome.

While no single cause can be defined, possible mediating mechanisms include 1) damage to spermatozoa, 2) the presence of the drug or its metabolites in the seminal fluid, 3) other alterations in semen, and 4) indirect effects resulting from endocrine, behavioral, and other effects on the sire.

In summary, to date little attention has been focused on the effect of chemical agents ingested by the father on his progeny. The results of our studies, together with those reported in the literature, suggest that such effects may be a general pharmacologic phenomenon. While additional studies are urgently needed to elucidate the underlying mechanism(s) of action and to define the clinical significance, if any, of such paternally mediated drug effects, it seems possible that studies in this field may introduce a new dimension to our concepts of reproductive biology.

ACKNOWLEDGMENTS

Studies were supported in part by NIDA 01160. Mrs. Sue M. Smith and Mr. John M. Peterson provided technical support. Ms. Mary Jane J. Dodds assisted in preparation of the manuscript.

REFERENCES

1. Smith DJ, Joffe JM. Nature 253:202, 1975.
2. Joffe JM, Peterson JM, Smith DJ, Soyka LF. Res Commun Chem Pathol Pharmacol 13: 611, 1976.
3. Soyka LF, Peterson JM, Joffe JM. Toxicol Appl Pharmacol 45:797, 1978.
4. Soyka LF, Joffe JM, Peterson JM, Smith SM. Pharmacol Biochem Behav 9:409, 1978.
5. Epstein SS, Röhrborn G. Nature 230:459, 1971.
6. Soyka LF, Joffe JM, Smith SM. Develop Pharmacol Ther, submitted.
7. Joffe JM. Clin Perinatol 6:21, 1979.
8. Cole LJ, Bachhuber LJ. Proc Soc Exp Biol Med 12:24, 1914.
9. Weller CV. J Med Res 33:271, 1915.
10. Stowe HD, Goyer RA. Fertil Steril 22:755, 1971.
11. Brady K, Herrera Y, Zenick H. Pharmacol Biochem Behav 3:561, 1975.
12. Friedler G. Fed Proc 33:515, 1974.
13. Stockard CR. Am Nat 47:641, 1913.
14a. MacDowell EC, Lord EM, MacDowell CG. Proc Soc Exp Biol Med 23:517, 1926.
14b. MacDowell EC, Lord EM, MacDowell CG. Proc Soc Exp Biol Med 23:652, 1926.
14c. MacDowell EC, Lord EM. Arch Entwickl Org 110:427, 1927.
15. Durham FM, Woods HM. Med Res Counc Spec Rep Ser No 168 (London), 1932.
16. Badr FM, Badr RS. Nature 253:134, 1975.
17. Klassen RW, Persaud TVN. Exp Pathol Bd 12:38, 1976.
18. Weathersbee PS, Ax RL, Lodge JR. J Reprod Fertil 43:141, 1975.
19. Lutwak-Mann C. Br Med J 1:1090, 1964.
20. Pearl R. J Exp Zool 22:241, 1917.
21. Ax RL, Lodge JR. Ill Res 18:18, 1976.
22. Dalldorf G, Williams RR. Science 102:668, 1945.
23. Morris HP, Lang EP, Morris HJ, Grant RL. J Pharmacol Exp Ther 64:420, 1938.

24. Paul C. Arch Gen Med 1:513, 1860. (Quoted by Weller [9].)
25. Chyzzer A. Chir Presse (Budapest) 44:906, 1908 (Quoted by Weller [9]).
26. Rudeaux, P. La Clinique (Jan. 21, 1910). Quoted by Thompson. "The Occupational Diseases." Appleton and Co., 1914, p 234.
27. Reid G. Report of the Department Commission on the dangers attendant on the use of lead. Quoted by T. Oliver. Br Med J 1:1096, 1911.
28. Ad Hoc Committee on the effect of trace anesthetics on the health of operating room personnel. Anesthesiology 41:321, 1974.
29. Cohen EN, Brown BW Jr, Bruce DL, Cascorbi HF, Corbett TH, Jones TW, Whitcher CE. J Am Dent Assoc 90:1291, 1975.
30. Yerushalmy J. Am J Epidemiol 93:443, 1971.
31. Weathersbee PS, Olsen LK, Lodge JR. Postgrad Med 62:64, 1977.
32. Soyka LF, Joffe JM, Peterson JM, Smith SM. Pediatr Res 12:409, 1978.
33. Falek A, Jordan RB, King BJ, Arnold PJ, Skelton WD. Arch Gen Psychiatry 27:511, 1972.
34. Friedler G, Wurster-Hill D. Proc 36th Annual Meeting of Committee on Problems of Drug Dependence, Mexico City, 1974.
35. Lutwak-Mann C, Schmid K, Keberle H. Nature 214:1018, 1967.
36. Gerber N, Lynn RK. Life Sci 19:787, 1976.
37. Swanson BN, Leger RJ, Gordon WP, Lynn RK, Gerber N. Drug Metab Dispos 6:70, 1978.
38. Peterson RN, Freund M. Biol Reprod 13:552, 1975.
39. Christiansen P, Dergaard J, Lund M. Ugeskr Laeger 137:2402, 1975.
40. Cicero TJ, Bell RD, Wiest WG, Allison JH, Polanski K, Robbins E. N Engl J Med 292:882, 1975.
41. Ericsson RJ, Baker VF. J Reprod Fertil 12:381, 1966.
42. Macht DI. J Pharmacol Exp Ther 10:509, 1918.
43. Hartman CG. Ann NY Acad Sci 83:318, 1959.
44. Paladine WJ, Cunningham TJ, Donovan MA, Dumper CW. N Engl J Med 292:52, 1975.
45. Cicero TJ, Meyer ER, Wiest WG, Olney JW, Bell RD. J Pharnacol Exp Ther 192:542, 1975.
46. Karim SMM (ed): The Prostaglandins. In "Progress in Research." New York: Wiley, 1972.
47. Cicero TJ, Wilcox CE, Bell RD, Meyer ER. J Pharnacol Exp Ther 198:340, 1961.
48. Cicero TJ, Meyer ER, Bell RD, Koch GA. Endocrinology 98:367, 1976.
49. Cicero TJ, Meyer ER. J Pharmacol Exp Ther 184:404, 1973.
50. Cicero TJ, Meyer ER, Bell RD, Wiest WG. Res Commun Chem Pathol Pharmacol 7:17, 1974.
51. Cicero TJ, Bell RD, Meyer ER, Schweitzer J. J Pharmacol Exp Ther 201:76, 1977.
52. Cushman Jr. P Am J Med 55:452, 1973.
53. Mendelson JH, Mendelson JE, Patch VD. Fed Proc 33:232, 1974.
54. Mendelson JH, Inturrisi CE, Renault P, Senay EG. Clin Pharmacol Ther 19:371, 1976.
55. Kreek MJ. JAMA 223:6, 1973.
56. Wilson JR, Adler N, LeBoeuf B. Proc Natl Acad Sci USA 53:1392, 1965.
57. Adler NT, Resko JA, Goy RW. Physiol Behav 5:1003, 1970.
58. Adler NT, Zoloth SR. Science 168:1480, 1970.

Drug and Other Hazards to the Fetus and Newborn

Martha M. Freeman, MD, and Marion J. Finkel, MD

FDA is responsible for ensuring that marketed drugs have an acceptable benefit-to-risk ratio for their intended uses, and that they are adequately labeled to permit them to be administered safely and effectively. In meeting this responsibility, it has long been concerned with the effects on the unborn child and neonate of drugs to which the pregnant woman is exposed. In addition, FDA has been concerned about the effect of food additives, cosmetics, and pesticides. I will confine this discussion, however, mainly to its activities in the drug area.

FDA's investigational new drug regulations, supplemented by its clinical guidelines, require that, with few exceptions, a new drug not be administered to women capable of becoming pregnant until preliminary stuides have been performed in pregnant animals, and reasonable evidence of the drug's clinical safety and effectiveness has been demonstrated in men, and in women not capable of childbearing. This emphasis on fetal safety is not surprising in view of the fact that the regulations were developed to implement the Kefauver-Harris Amendments to the Food, Drug and Cosmetic Act, which were enacted by the Congress in 1962 in the prevailing climate of societal concerns generated by the thalidomide episode in Europe. Until that time, under the existing FD&C Act of 1938, the requirement that drugs be cleared for safety prior to marketing had been intrepreted primarily in terms of acute and chronic toxicity data from animal studies and the defining of adverse effects in human subjects. Even at that time, however, FDA was becoming increasingly aware of environmental hazards to the fetus. In addition to the recognition in 1929 of adverse effects on the fetus of x-radiation in early pregnancy, and in 1941 of rubella virus-induced congenital malformations, there were also reports in the early 1940s of animal and clinical studies demonstrating that the fetus and newborn metabolize drugs differently, both qualitatively and quantitatively, than adults, and they are, therefore, potentially at greater risk of adverse effects from drugs. The significance of their undeveloped enzyme systems was demonstrated by the unique toxicity of chloramphenicol in premature infants reported in 1958.

Drug and Chemical Risks to the Fetus and Newborn: 67–72

One of the first drugs recognized to have a teratogenic potential was aminopterin, which was marketed in 1951 for treatment of acute leukemia. Since abortifacient effects had been noted in animals, the labeling bore a strong warning that folic antagonists had been shown to have adverse effects on the embryo in experimental animals and therefore should not be used in pregnancy. Subsequently aminopterin's teratogenic effect in humans was demonstrated by reports of severely malfored children born to mothers who had received the drug for attempted therapeutic or criminal abortion. The thalidomide episode in the early 1960s provided compelling evidence that, unless proven otherwise, chemical and physical agents must be seriously regarded as having a potential for adverse effects on the human fetus.

Following the 1962 drug law amendments, attention was directed primarily toward malformations induced by teratogenic substances during critical early periods of organogenesis. More recently concern has been extended to possible delayed adverse effects of agents administered during various stages of pregnancy, labor, and delivery, including neurobehavioral, mutagenic, and carcinogenic effects in the offspring. There is also increasing awareness of the vulnerability of the fetus and the neonate to the pharmacologic effects of maternally administered drugs which themselves produce no adverse effects in the mothers; examples include protracted hypoglycemia from oral antidiabetic agents and goiter from iodide-containing preparations.

FDA policy and programs relative to fetal protection have developed along two lines: 1) the testing requirements to establish safety and effectiveness of new products for marketing, and 2) the surveillance of the products aftery they are marketed in order to detect previously unsuspected adverse effects and delayed or long-term effects, and to determine the incidence of known adverse effects.

Before a new drug substance can be introduced into man, safety data must be submitted by the manufacturer, including chemical control information, the results of animal toxicity studies, the results of foreign experience if the drug has been used outside the United States, and a reasonable plan for studying the drug in humans. With few exceptions, animal reproduction studies in at least one species and teratology studies in at least two species must be carried out before involving women of childbearing potential as subjects. The current FDA guidelines for reproduction studies in animals are designed to determine effects of drugs on the entire reproductive process, including the effects on fertility in the male and female, on conception and implantation in the uterus, on development and survival of the fetus, on the birth process, on the quantity and quality of the maternal milk supply, and on the survival of the offspring.

If animal studies show no adverse effects on the reproductive spectrum, or, at least, no effects until very large doses are given, and clinical pharmacologic and early clinical studies in males and postmenopausal women have shown reasonable safety and effectiveness, women of childbearing potential may then be included in clinical trials. It is important, however, that the informed consent procedure (which is required for all investigational subjects) should include information on the animal reproduction studies and clearly specify that such studies cannot, however, ensure safety for the human fetus. If a woman's health needs require it, even teratogenic drugs may be administered with her informed consent. In either case, inadvertent fetal recipients should be followed throughout the pregnancy and carefully examined for abnormalities at birth and at one year.

Testing drugs in women who are known to be pregnant poses complex ethical problems that are not yet resolved. Only those few drugs intended for treating conditions specifically related to pregnancy justify controlled clinical trials in pregnant women to determine safety for the mother and unborn child and effectiveness in the mother. It is not feasible to assess prior to marketing the safety for the human fetus of the majority of prescription drugs used for treating diseases that occur in both prgenant and nonpregnant patients, even though physicians are free to prescribe such drugs, once marketed, for women of childbearing potential. Cognizant of this dilemma, FDA requires that labeling information for all drugs provide, in a concise form, all pertinent data on animal reproduction studies and any known adverse effects on the human fetus. In the near future FDA will also require that the labeling describe any adequate human experience based upon well-controlled studies or epidemiologic studies that demonstrates the safety of drugs for the human fetus. All of this information allows the physician and his pregnant patient to select the drug best suited to her needs with least risk to her unborn child.

Surveillance of drugs, once marketed, for damaging effects on the fetus is not readily accomplished through voluntary reporting of adverse effects by physicians. Although many physicians do report to the FDA congenital anomalies in offspring of women who received various drugs during pregnancy, unless a striking and rare anomaly, such as phocomelia, is observed in association with a drug, more structured types of surveillance, that is epidemiologic surveys, both retrospective and prospective, are required to establish a relationship between a drug and congenital malformations.

For drugs of limited use but critical to small patient populations, patient registries can also be established to permit prospective monitoring for possible teratogenic and other adverse effects. As new information becomes available its significance is evaluated by FDA, and the drug's benefit to risk ratio is reassessed, frequently in conjunction with FDA's advisory committees. If it is determined that the hazards outweigh a drug's benefit, it may be removed from the market. Where the risks are less serious, labeling may be revised to provide for more limited indications and additional warning information. Physicians and health professionals are informed of these actions and the reasons for them through FDA's Drug Bulletin. They are also publicized through press releases and the FDA Consumer Magazine. FDA is also initiating a program of patient informational leaflets for most drugs.

At present these leaflets are required primarily for drugs the use of which is significantly or wholly elective in nature and which are associated with serious risks – namely, the oral contraceptives, estrogens and progestational agents. In addition to describing the potential carcinogenicity and other serious effects of estrogenic products in women, the known potential of the estrogens and progestagens for causing serious malformations in the fetus is discussed in the leaflets.

Current animal teratological methodology is effective in providing meaningful data on the teratogenic potential of chemicals in the conventional sense – that is the gross observation of congenital anomalies. To ensure that all scientific data gathered during these studies are most effectively employed, a selected analysis of chemicals for which there is definitive human and animal teratology information is being performed by FDA. This effort will help resolve some questions concerning the correlation of teratogenic effects in animals with the potential for such effects in humans.

In addition, existing laboratory data bases will be examined to determine dose-response curves in order to permit the development or identification of appropriate biomathematical procedures for low dose risk estimation for teratogens.

The potential for maternally administered drugs to cause functional and developmental impairment in the offspring has been recognized for some time, but current guidelines for reproductive and conventional teratology testing do not address the issue directly. A few European countries and Japan now have very general requirements for behavioral teratology testing; and the recently enacted Toxic Substances Control Act mandates such testing in the United States for chemicals under the jurisdiction of the Environmental Protection Agency. Yet the basic information concerning validity and relevance of testing procedures has not been assembled. In fact the present state of the art in the field of behavioral teratology testing is such that, in our opinion, it is not scientifically credible to perform large-scale testing in the absence of assurance that it would yield meaningful data. The FDA, through its National Center for Toxicological Research (NCTR) is initiating steps to develop valid screening methods in this field. Experts from academia, industry, and the government will select four to six behavioral test methods that appear to have the greatest potential utility in screening, develop standardized protocols, and oversee their study by several contractual laboratories. The data will be collated from each test procedure and interlaboratory comparisons made. Upon completion of the entire project (approximately three years in duration), the data will be presented at a conference, and recommendations will be made concerning the incorporation of behavioral teratology methods into reproduction and teratology testing guidelines. In this way the responsibility for developing adequate testing procedures and influencing regulatory policy will be that of the scientific community at large.

While these various studies are ongoing, FDA must continue to regulate drugs on the basis of the best available information. The Collaborative Perinatal Project of the National Institute of Neurological and Communicative Disorders and Stroke appears to offer a fertile source for data on drug effects. This prospective study involved approximately 50,000 pregnant women and their offspring entered between 1959 and 1965 with a structured follow-up of the offspring to the age of eight. It was designed to identify factors in pregnancy related to cerebral palsy and other forms of central nervous system damage, but it also lends itself to analysis of other congenital anomalies and neurobehavioral disorders. The study obtained information on drug intake of the mothers throughout pregnancy and delivery. FDA provided contractual support for a detailed analysis of drug intake during the first four months of pregnancy and pregnancy outcome. A book titled "Birth Defects and Drugs in Pregnancy" by Heinonen et al ensued. The findings of Heinonen and co-workers supported the suspected association between certain drugs and congenital anomalies and raised hypotheses requiring further testing of other drugs. A definitive analysis of the drugs used in labor and delivery and infant outcome is expected in 1982. Although the latter analysis may shed some light on long-term effects on the neurological development of the offspring, one drawback of the study is that it is limited to drugs marketed prior to 1965, and to obstretrical practices many of which have been superseded in the past 15 years. Within the past year there has been considerable publicity in the media of a preliminary unpublished analysis of a subset of the data involving drugs given during labor and delivery. This analysis purported to demonstrate that the effects of perinatal exposure to thse drugs persist into childhood, causing developmental delays and impaired behavior and intelligence. The publicity resulted in considerable anxiety on the part of women and criticism in the scientific community that the report had not been subjected to peer review. Because of the public concern on the matter, in March 1979 FDA convened a panel of experts in anesthesiology, neurology, obstetrics, developmental pediatrics, biostatistics, and epidemiology to review and discuss with the authors the unpublished report, plus all pertinent published data on the subject of neurobehavioral effects in the newborn of drugs administered during labor and delivery. FDA also asked the panel to advise it on whether any action relative to the drugs is warranted at this time and to advise as to what additional types of studies, if any, should be required to market new drugs for labor and delivery. The panel advised that the available published data do suggest that perinatal drugs are associated with short-term neurological effects in newborns, and that present labeling in this regard is adequate. They further advised that, due to flaws in the analysis of the unpublished data on long-term effects, valid conclusions cannot be reached pending further review by a specially appointed subcommittee. The panel also supported the position of The American Academy of Pediatrics and the American College of Obstretrics and Gynecology that perinatal drug exposure be kept to a minimum consistent with good medical practice and that the lowest effective doses be employed.

Although this discussion has focused on drugs, similar considerations apply to medical devices and the effects of radiation and ultrasound. For example, increasing concern has arisen regarding the fetal safety of widely used diagnostic ultrasound in obstretrics. Animal studies have been reported to reveal delayed neuromuscular development, altered emotional behavior, EEG changes, anomalies, and decreased survival. Genetic alterations have also been demonstrated in in vitro systems. Whether any of these findings can be extrapolated to humans is not known at this time. FDA is now funding a retrospective epidemiologic study designed to compare the physical and behavioral development in 1,600 offspring exposed in utero to ultrasound, and 1,600 non-exposed controls. Until definitive data are available in humans to support valid conclusions, FDA has taken the position recommended by its Obstetrical and Gynecological Device Classification Panel that ultrasound should be used only when there is a valid medical indication and confined to the lowest exposure levels consistent with obtaining essential diagnostic information. It should be noted that ultrasound exposure of pregnant women for commercial demonstration of equipment is not considered acceptable by most professional organizations in the field.

Considerable research remains to be done to evaluate the risks to the fetus of drugs, other chemicals, and devices. It will always be considered prudent, however, to avoid unnecessary exposure. At the same time the public must recognize that, in the interests of the mother, necessary exposure should not be avoided. It is important that pregnant women receive available information on drugs and devices to which they may be exposed and that they participate with their physicians in the decision to use these agents.

Alcohol Effects on the Fetus

David W. Smith, MD

We are now into the era of fetal medicine.* Most of the handicapping disorders of infants and children we care for today are the consequence of problems in prenatal development. Though the majority of these problems appear to have a genetic basis, it is extremely important to recognize those that have an environmental etiology since they are more readily preventable. When a chemical agent becomes recognized as causing problems in fetal development – ie, as being teratogenic – every attempt should be made to prevent the exposure of the fetus to dangerous levels of that chemical agent. This information should reach all women of reproductive age who are receiving the teratogen or who are liable to receive it after conception.

Mothering before birth is direct mothering. It is direct in the sense that most chemical agents that the mother takes during pregnancy are also "taken" by the fetus.

If we can simply foster the concept of *mothering from conception,* this will be a major philosophical advance toward prenatal preventive medicine. For example, every women needs to know that her cigarette smoking or alcohol ingestion is cigarette smoking or alcohol ingestion by the fetus. Just as she would not wish her infant to smoke or drink after birth, it is even more important that the fetus not be exposed before birth, by her own smoking or drinking. All women who are chronically taking certain teratogenic medications such as hydantoins need to know the risk to the developing fetus, and attempts should be made to avoid the risk. The nature and magnitude of risks for all of the more readily accessible agents that are considered teratogenic in the human have been

*I have taken the liberty of using the term "fetus," which is Latin for "offspring" or "young one," to encompass the entire period of prenatal life, including the embryonic period.

This has recently been published by the American Academy of Pediatrics in Smith, D.W.: Fetal Drug Syndromes; Effects of Ethanol and Hydantoins. Pediatrics in Review 1: 1979.

Drug and Chemical Risks to the Fetus and Newborn: 73–82

set forth in a book for the lay public titled "Mothering Your Unborn Baby" [1]. A more complete medical catalogue of teratogenic agents has been published by Shepard [2].

This paper will discuss ethanol as to the most common teratogen, aside from cigarette smoking, to which fetuses are being exposed today.

But first a few thoughts about teratogens in general, thoughts that are applicable to both ethanol and hydantoins. I use alcohol as an example, but the precepts also apply to hydantoins. First, the impact of a given teratogen can seldom be predicted from its effects on the mature individual. For example, ethanol has toxic consequences on the adult, but these effects have not provided a rationale for understanding the effects of ethanol on the developing fetus. Thus ethanol may cause liver cirrhosis in the adult, but the liver is seldom one of the fetal tissues that is affected.

Second, the teratogenic effect may be due to the ingested agent or to one of its breakdown products. At present the question remains open whether the fetal alcohol syndrome is due to ethanol or to its breakdown product, acetaldehyde.

Third, the most common impact of known teratogens in man is a pattern of malformation. Though individual features of the malformation pattern are nonspecific, the overall pattern has specificity. The recognition of a rather concise syndrome allows for a more thorough detection of causal factors in different individuals with the same syndrome. Thus, the detection of a unique pattern of malformation among the offspring of chronically alcoholic women identified ethanol (or its degradation product) as a human teratogen.

However, it is very dangerous to limit one's thinking to the more complete pattern of malformation. A teratogen tends to give rise to a spectrum of defects, a spectrum that may vary greatly both in extent and severity. Thus as exemplified in Figure 1, one observes all gradations – from normal, to mildly affected, to moderately affected, to the full spectrum of the fetal alcohol syndrome – in individuals exposed to heavy maternal ethanol intake in utero. Among the affected children the questions should not be "Does the child have the fetal alcohol syndrome?"; rather, the question should be "Is the child's problem secondary to alcohol exposure in utero?"

Fourth, a teratogen seldom causes defects in 100% of exposed fetuses. Obviously, the timing of maternal ingestion is a factor. Beyond this consideration, the impact of the agent depends on the level of intake by the mother, her capability for degrading the agent, the ability of the fetus to metabolize the teratogen, and the response of the fetal tissues to the agent. Genetic differences in the mother and in the fetus can modulate the relative impact of a given intake of a teratogen.

Finally, once a particular agent is identified as a teratogen, it is usually difficult to state a "safe dose" for the fetus. At the milder level of severity, the effects may be quite difficult to detect, according to studies on small numbers of ex-

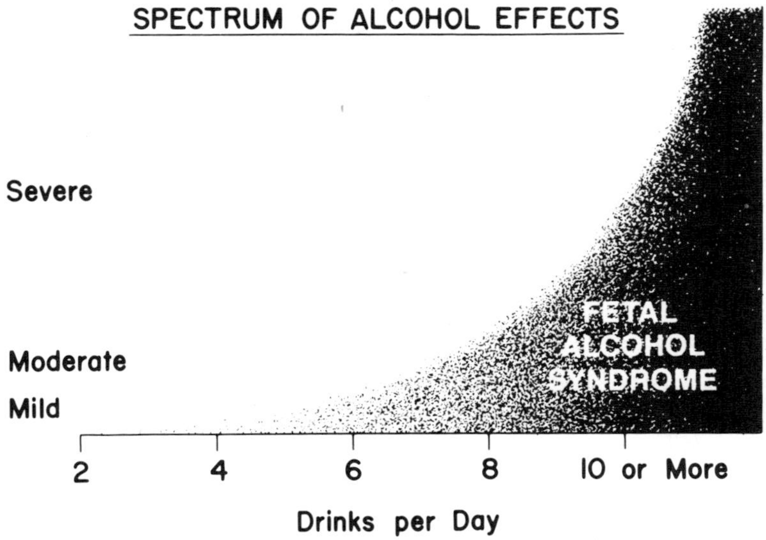

Fig. 1. The spectrum of potential alcohol effects on the fetus range from very mild to severe in degree and extent. The fetal alcohol syndrome represents the most severe end of the spectrum and commonly occurs in women who are chronically alcoholic. By Ms Jan Norbisrath, Department of Obstetrics and Gynecology, University of Washington Medical School.

posed individuals. At what level of ethanol exposure is there an average drop of five points in IQ? This would be most difficult to determine. Furthermore, there has been no teratogen yet studied in man that clearly shows a threshold effect, with the substance being quite safe to a particular level, beyond which it is teratogenic.

FETAL ALCOHOL EFFECTS, INCLUDING FETAL ALCOHOL SYNDROME

Historical

The serious impact of alcohol on fetal development was independently implied in 1834, in the 1880s, the early 1900s, and by Ulleland in 1972 [3]. The broader clinical features of the fetal alcohol syndrome were independently set forth in France by Rouquette in 1957 [4] and again by Lemoine in 1968 [5]. Unfortunately, the serious implications in each of these reports did not become general medical or public knowledge. Lemoine later wrote to me that his observations "were never accepted by my colleagues." Hence in 1972, ethanol was not generally considered to be a human teratogen. Following the reports in 1973 of Jones and co-workers [6] about the fetal alcohol syndrome, there has been an ever-increasing recognition that ethanol is the most common chemical teratogen causing problems of malformation and mental deficiency in the human [7–10]. I am aware of at least 618 affected individuals, including groups of 85 or more patients in Seattle, Vancouver, Nantes (France), and Tübingen (Germany), centers where one or more investigator has had a specific interest in this disorder, in regions where heavy alcohol intake during pregnancy is not rare. Studies in Seattle and in France have disclosed an incidence of fetal alcohol syndrome of more than one per thousand live births. The prospective Seattle study of Hanson et al [10] indicated a 0.2% frequency of fetal alcohol syndrome, and an additional 0.4% frequency of newborn babies showing less severe degrees of alcohol effect.

Clinical Features

There is a wide range of variability in the spectrum of effects on the fetus. The least impact which has been documented, so mild that it may be questioned, is the effect of two drinks per day.* At this level of exposure babies have averaged 60–160 gm smaller than expected at birth [11]. No major fetal effects have been noted at an intake of less than four drinks per day [8]. The various features of the fetal alcohol syndrome have been predominatly observed in the children of women taking four to six or more drinks per day, and especially in the offspring of chronically alcoholic women.

The most consistent effects of heavy alcohol exposure to the fetus have been growth deficiency, brain dysfunction, and subtle facial dysmorphia, as summarized in Figure 2. These constitute the predominant features of the fetal alcohol syndrome, but there are also a host of nonrandomly occurring malformations in this syndrome.

Growth. Prenatal growth deficiency for weight, length, and head circumference is frequent. There is seldom any catch-up growth postnatally; in fact, the children tend to become underweight for height during infancy and childhood, with diminished adipose tissue. Thus they may be misinterpreted as representing "failure-to-thrive" of postnatal onset.

Brain and its dysfunction. Brain growth is liable to be even more deficient than linear or weight growth. All gradations of mental deficiency have been noted, with IQs from 16 to 105, with an average of 65 for children with fetal alcohol syndrome. Fine motor coordination is often poor, and hypotonia may be a feature. Affected individuals tend to be fretful in infancy and hyperative in mid-childhood.

Facial dysmorphia. The facies often have a distinctive appearance as shown in Figure 3. The palpebral fissures tend to be short, possibly because the eye size is small. The nose may be somewhat small and short, with a low nasal bridge and redundant inner canthal skin folds. Short nose may give the philtral region the appearance of being long. The philtrum tends to be smooth and as a con-

*One drink is the equivalent of one whiskey, one beer, or one medium glass of wine.

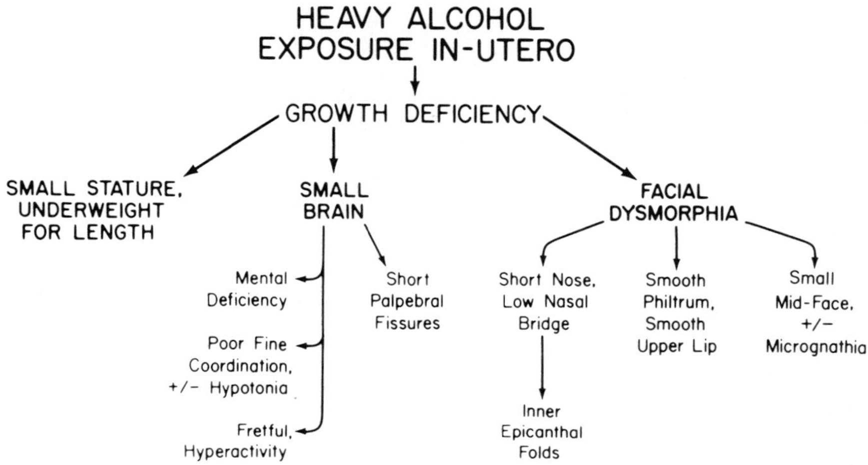

Fig. 2. The most consistent features that occur in individuals with the fetal alcohol syndrome may be interpreted as the consequence of dysharmonic growth deficiency. By Ms Jan Norbisrath, Department of Obstetrics and Gynecology, University of Washington Medical School.

sequence the upper lip may lack its usual indentation bow. The vermillion of the upper lip may be thin. The maxilla tend to be a bit small, especially as growth progresses. The mandible may also be small. Hirsutism may be notable at birth and usually recedes postnatally.

Other malformations. Table I lists the other malformations that have occurred with increased frequency in children with the fetal alcohol syndrome [9]. There is hardly an organ tissue or body system that has not been affected. It is very important to appreciate that many patients with fetal alcohol syndrome are evaluated by a physician primarily because of a major malformation. Hence the neurologist, the cardiologist, the urologist, the ophthalmologist, and a variety of other specialists should be alert to the malformations of their subspecialty interest that occur as one feature of the fetal alcohol syndrome.

Withdrawal effects after birth can include irritibility, tremulousness and, occassionally, transient seizures. The withdrawl phenomenon, when present, is usually not a serious problem.

Differential diagnosis. There is no single feature of the fetal alcohol syndrome that is pathognomonic, and there are a number of other disorders that share some of the same features, including the fetal hydantoin syndrome. The most common prior misdiagnoses for patients with the fetal alcohol syndrome have been de Lange syndrome, Noonan syndrome, and Williams syndrome [12]. A rare autosomal recessive disorder, Dubowitz syndrome, is very similar to the fetal alcohol syndrome. Also the total diagnosis has often been missed in a fetal

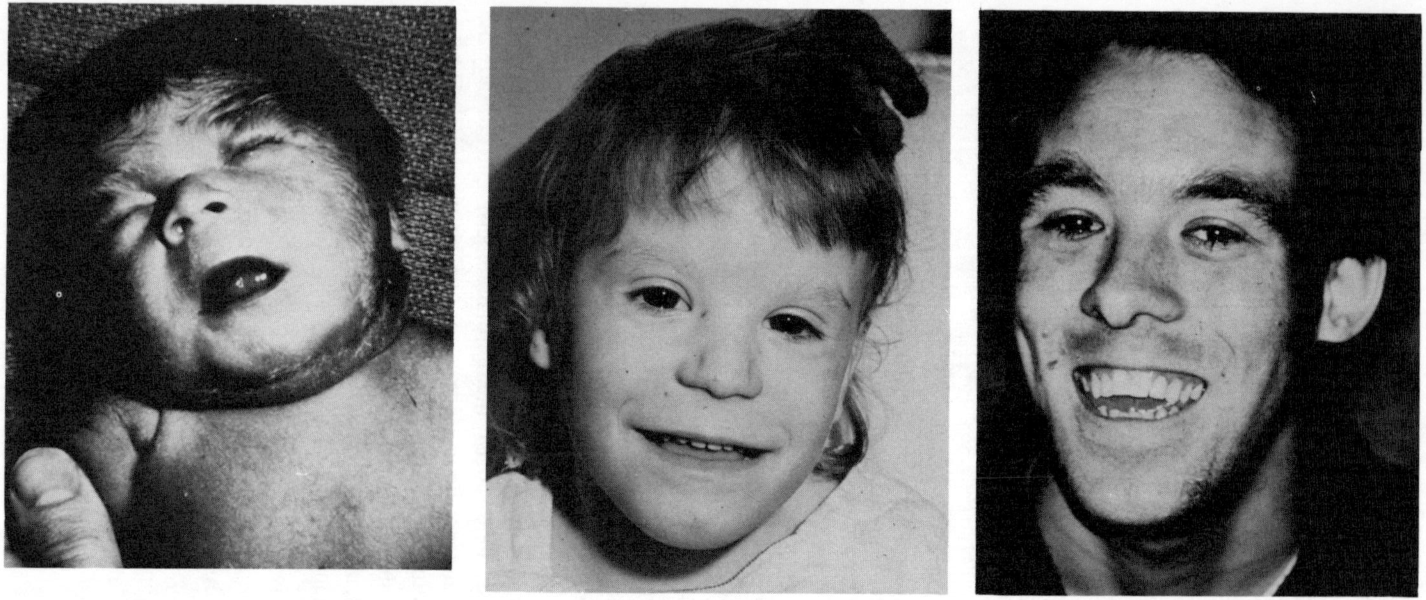

Fig. 3. Facial features of the fetal alcohol syndrome. Left: Infant at birth. Middle: Child at 4 years of age. Right: 22-year-old. Note hirsutism at birth, the short palpebral fissures, poor philtrum with smooth upper lip, plus variable small maxilla with age, strabismus, mild ptosis, minor ear anomaly, and relatively small nose. Left and middle are from Hanson JW, Jones KL, Smith DW: Fetal alcohol syndrome. JAMA 235:1548, 1978. Right photo is from Clarren SK, Smith DW: The fetal alcohol syndrome. N Engl J Med 298:1063, 1978.

TABLE I. Non-Random Defects Noted in Children With Fetal Alcohol Syndrome

Areas	Relatively frequent (26–50%)	Occasionals (1–25%)
Nervous system		Meningomyelocele, hydrocephalus
Eyes	Strabismus, ptosis	Myopia, gross microphthalmia
Ears	Protruding auricle	Poorly formed concha
Mouth	Prominent lateral palatine ridges	Cleft lip, cleft palate
Cardiac	Atrial septal defect	Ventricular septal defect, tetralogy of Fallot, great vessel anomalies
Genitourinary	Labial hypoplasia	Renal malformation, hypospadias
Skin	Hemangiomata	Hirsutism in infancy
Hands	Unusual palmar creases	Clinodactyly 5th fingers, camptodactyly, hypoplastic nails, esp. 5th, syndactyly 3rd–4th fingers
Skeletal		Elbow limitation, synostosis, cervical vertebral anomalies, pectus excavatum or carinatum, bifid xyphoid
Other		Hernia of diaphragm, umbilicus, groin diastasis recti

alcohol syndrome patient with a major malformation because there is a tendency to focus on the major malformation rather than on the total pattern of malformation, which includes growth and mental deficiency.

Pathogenesis. As depicted in Figure 2, much of the dysmorphia caused by heavy ethanol exposure in utero may be interpreted as the consequence of dysharmonic growth deficiency yielding a diminished cell number, which is more profound in some tissues than in others. However, the developmental pathology may also include faulty cell migration in brain morphogenesis [13]. Animal studies have now experimentally reproduced the features of the fetal alcohol syndrome. They have demonstrated that the severity of the effects on the fetus relates to the level of blood ethanol achieved in the pregnant mother. Furthermore, the impact has clearly been related to ethanol intake and not to secondary malnutrition in the alcoholized animal.

The question remains whether the teratogenic molecule is ethanol itself or its breakdown product, acetaldehyde. This question merits further resolution.

Another potential variable is the response of the individual fetus to ethanol. Ethanol readily crosses the placenta into all fetal tissues, but we do not know the fetal capacities for degrading ethanol and/or acetaldehyde. We have had experience with dizygotic twins born of an alcoholic mother: One twin had features of fetal alcohol syndrome at birth, whereas the other was physically normal. This implies individual variability in the fetal response to ethanol.

Risk Counsel

The risk of a serious problem in the offspring of chronically alcoholic women has been estimated to be in the range of 30–50% [7].

We know that heavy exposure to ethanol may cause serious problems during the first trimester. For example, we recently evaluated an eight-year-old boy whose mother had been alcoholic but stopped her alcohol consumption completely during the fourth month of pregnancy. The child has a typical facies and multiple features of the fetal alcohol syndrome. We do not have adequate data on the effects of heavy alcohol exposure during the second trimester alone or the third trimester only.

It is not possible to state a safe level of alcohol exposure by the fetus; it is quite easy, however, to state that the ideal is no ethanol exposure. As previously indicated, the least intake at which a measurable fetal effect has been appreciated has been the equivalent of two drinks per day [11]. We do not have ideal data for the risk at a given level of alcohol intake. At present the best guide is a prospective study on the offspring of 1,500 women by Hanson et al [10] which showed partial features of the fetal alcohol syndrome in 11% of offspring whose mothers consumed two to four drinks per day and 19% in offspring of those drinking four or more drinks per day. In that study there were three women who drank ten or more drinks per day, each of whom would be classed as chronically alcoholic, and all three offspring were considered to have the fetal alcohol syndrome. These data again implicate a spectrum of increasing severity and risk with increasing alcohol intake by the pregnant woman.

Prevention

"Behold, thou shalt conceive, and bear a son; and now drink no wine or strong drink. . . ." (Judges 13:7).

This biblical statement has relevance today. The effects of alcohol on the fetus are totally preventable. The knowledge of the effects of alcohol on the fetus should become general public knowledge. Just as a woman would not wish her infant to drink alcohol after birth, so she must appreciate that the fetus shares the alcohol she consumes, as depicted in Figure 1, and that the most dangerous period for exposure to high levels of alcohol is during fetal life.

It is of utmost importance that any women of reproductive age who is chronically alcoholic know the risk. Ideally such a woman should be on birth control measures and should have the option of terminating any pregnancy that occurs while she is alcoholic.

The nature and magnitude of the fetal risks from moderate maternal alcohol consumption need to be further studied, as does the impact of heavy binge drinking at a given time during gestation. Until reasonably clear answers are available, the safest approach is to limit alcohol consumption during pregnancy.

COMMENT

Having become familiar with the fetal alcohol syndrome, I have been increasingly impressed by the number of children who have less severe partial features of the disorder. No longer is the question "Does a child have fetal alcohol syndrome?"; rather, the question is, "Is this child's problem secondary to alcohol exposure in utero?" This becomes a judgmental question, largely based on the experience of the clinician. The "possible alcohol effect" patients may derive from a chronically alcoholic mother, but may also derive from a moderately heavy (four to eight drinks a day) or an intermittent binge drinking mother. In contrast, the fetal alcohol syndrome patient has usually been born to a chronically alcoholic woman.

ACKNOWLEDGMENTS

The major contributions of Drs. Kenneth L. Jones, James W. Hanson, and Sterling K. Clarren, former dysmorphology fellows, are gratefully appreciated, as is the assistance of Ms Lyle Harrah, Mary Ann Sedgwick Harvey, Jane Fowler, and Jill Wolcott.

This work was supported by Bureau of Community Health Services, Health Services Administration, Public Health Service, Department of Health, Education and Welfare Project 913, National Institutes of Health grant HD 05961, Public Health Service grant GM 15253.

REFERENCES

1. Smith DW: "Mothering Your Unborn Child." Philadelphia: WB Saunders, 1979.
2. Shepard TH (ed): "Catalog of Teratogenic Agents, Ed 2. Baltimore: The Johns Hopkins University Press, 1976.
3. Ulleland CN: The offspring of alcoholic mothers. Ann NY Acad Sci 197:167, 1972.
4. Rouquette J: Influence of parental alcoholic toxemia on the physical and psychological development of young children. Thesis for Doctorate of Medicine, University of Paris Faculty of Medicine, 1957.
5. Lemoine P, Harrousseau H, Borteyru JP, et al: Les enfants de parents alcooliques. Anomalies observées a propos de 127 cas. Ouest Med 21:476, 1968.
6. Jones KL, Smith DW, Ulleland N, et al: Pattern of malformation in offspring of chronic alcoholic mothers. Lancet 1:1267, 1973.

7. Jones KL, Smith, DW, Streissguth AP, et al: Outcome in offspring of chronic alcoholic women. Lancet 1:1076, 1974.
8. Majewski F, Bierich JR, Loser H, et al: Zur Klinik und Pathogenese der Alkohol-Embryo. Bericht uber 68 Falle. Munch Med Wochenschr 118:1635, 1976.
9. Clarren SK, Smith DW: The fetal alcohol syndrome: A review of the world literature. N Engl J Med 298:1063, 1978.
10. Hanson JW, Streissguth AP, Smith DW: The effects of moderate alcohol consumption during pregnancy on fetal growth and morphogenesis. J Pediatr 92:457, 1978.
11. Little R: Alcohol consumption during pregnancy and decreased birthweight. Am J Public Health 67:1154, 1977.
12. Smith DW: "Recognizable Patterns of Human Malformation," Ed 2. Philadelphia: WB Saunders, 1976.
13. Clarren SK, Alvord EC, Sumi SM, et al: Brain malformations related to prenatal exposure to alcohol. J Pediatr 92:64, 1978.
14. Chernoff GF: The fetal alcohol syndrome in mice: An animal model. Teratology 13:223, 1977.
15. Tze WJ, Leo M: Adverse effects of maternal alcohol consumption on pregnancy and foetal growth in rats. Nature 257:479, 2975.

Cigarettes and Pregnancy

Frank Witter, MD, and Theodore M. King, MD, PhD

INTRODUCTION

Since 1935 when Sontag first reported increased fetal heart rate with maternal smoking [1], the possibility of adverse effects of maternal smoking on the fetus has been under consideration. A large impetus to this interest was given by the Surgeon General's Report in 1964, which documented the adverse effects of smoking in the adult.

Present estimates are that the cigarette smoker has approximately 70% greater chance of dying from disease with an overall mortality ratio of 1.7 [2]. This excess mortality is due primarily to coronary heart disease, followed by lung cancer and chronic obstructive lung disease. Epidemiologic studies have related smoking to coronary heart disease, chronic bronchitis, emphysema, and to increased risk of thromboembolism in women who use oral contraceptives [2]. Smoking has also been related to myocardial infarction in women on oral contraceptives [3] and to a lower age for spontaneous menopause [4]. It has been associated with cancer of the lung, larynx, oral cavity, esophagus, stomach, pancreas, bladder, kidney, and uterine cervix [5]. In fact, if present increasing trends in mortality rates for lung cancer in women continue, lung cancer will be the leading cause of cancer deaths in women in the next decade [2].

Because of the adverse effects of smoking on the mother, the question of adverse effects on fetal growth and development must be addressed. This chapter reviews the evidence for the effects of smoking on the fetus.

FETAL GROWTH

The effect of smoking on fetal growth has been examined in many studies (Table I), and the most consistent finding that reflects an adverse effect is a decrease in birthweight of the infant [2,6–22]. This finding of decreased birthweight is consistent in these studies in spite of the diversity of the populations

Drug and Chemical Risks to the Fetus and Newborn: 83–92

TABLE I. Reduced Birthweight With Smoking

Source	Reduction in crude birthweight (gm)
Pirani et al [3]	138
Hardy and Nellis [9]	250
Bailey [10]	144–205
Butler et al [12]	170
Cope et al [17]	177
Yerushalmy [18] (white)	200
(black)	135

studied and, although there are a few who disagree [23,24], are attributable to smoking.

How smoking causes a decrease in birthweight has been a matter of debate. As weight gain also correlates with fetal growth, Rush [25] examined weight gain and correlated it with caloric intake. He found that smoking mothers showed a significant decrease in mean weekly weight gain, and that this decrease became more marked with increasing levels of maternal smoking. His conclusion was that the decreased fetal growth seen in smokers was due to the anorexic effect of smoking causing decreased caloric intake.

The thesis that decreased caloric intake due to smoking is the basis for reduced birthweights and maternal weight gain does not appear to be the answer. For Beal [19] in a longitudinal study of nutrition in pregnancy found that smoking mothers gave birth to infants with significantly lower mean birthweights despite higher average caloric intakes. In addition, Meyer [18,26], in an analysis of data from the Ontario Perinatal Mortality Study, showed that if the mothers were divided into groups according to weight gain, for each level of maternal weight gain the smoking mothers showed a greater percentage of infants weighing less than 2,500 grams and this percentage increased with increasing level of maternal smoking. The increase in infants under 2,500 grams was 20% for those smoking less than one pack per day and 340% for those smoking one pack or more per day. In addition, there was no significant difference in the distribution of maternal weight gain by smoking habit. The dose-response relation between level of smoking and birthweight has been confirmed by other studies [11,17,27].

Thus it appears that smoking produces its effect by other means than decreased caloric intake. To confirm this experimentally, rats were placed on a constant restricted caloric diet and exposed to cigarette smoke [16,27]. The rats exposed to cigarette smoke showed decreased fetal weight and decreased brain cell number when compared to controls.

Another possible explanation of the decreased birthweight in infants of smoking mothers is that smoking increases the incidence of premature birth. As prematurity is defined in some studies as birthweight less than 2,500 grams [7,25,27,28], this question is harder to answer. However, where gestational age was used as a criterion for prematurity, a significant increase was noted in some [6,18] but not all studies [2,19]. Smoking appears to act as an independent factor in decreasing birthweight [7,18] and to exert its deleterious effects after the fourth month, for if a mother decreases her smoking prior to the fourth month, her risk for decreased birthweight of her infant is decreased to the level of her new smoking status [15,29]. Buncher found that the average length of gestation in smoking mothers was decreased by 29 to 34 hours when compared to nonsmokers if they smoked one pack per day or more [30]. Further, he could attribute only about 10% of the known reduction in birthweight associated with smoking in pregnancy to this shortening of gestation.

Thus it appears that smoking produces significant intrauterine growth retardation [21]; however, Pirami [6] was unable to document any significant difference in urinary estriols, fetal biparietal diameter, and weekly growth rate, though the infants of smokers were significantly lighter. Naeye [31] studied women who smoked in one pregnancy but not in another and found that a lighter infant was produced in the pregnancy where the mother smoked, regardless of the birth order. How smoking produces its effect is not known, but there are several known components of cigarette smoke that could contribute. These components include carbon monoxide, nicotine, and cyanide.

The most extensively studied of these components is carbon monoxide. Carbon monoxide exerts its deleterious effect by decreasing fetal oxygenization. Hemoglobin has a high affinity for carbon monoxide – higher, in fact, than for oxygen [32]. Thus, the oxygenization of fetal blood decreases in direct proportion to the carboxyhemoglobin concentration in the maternal and fetal blood. Since fetal oxygen tension is normally 20–30% of the adult value, this decrease can result in severe hypoxia of vital tissues [33].

It has been shown that higher than normal maternal and cord blood levels of carboxyhemoglobin are present in smokers [27]. In fact, in a study of carboxyhemoglobin levels, Dow [34] showed a greater increase in carboxyhemoglobin concentration in response to smoking a single cigarette in the pregnant women (3.9% increase) than in the nonpregnant woman (2.1% increase). Further, this increase was greater with anemia (5.0% increase). Experimental confirmation that a higher than normal carbon monoxide level can, in and of itself, cause decreased birthweight is given by Fechter and Annau [35]. In their study, rats were exposed to low concentrations of carbon monoxide, which yielded carboxyhemoglobin levels equivalent to those in smokers and showed decreased weight gain and lower birthweight of their offspring.

Additional evidence that the effects of smoking are through decreased oxygen delivery to the fetus is given by Meyer and Tonascia [36] in their analysis of the Ontario Perinatal Mortality Study data. In their analysis they found an increase in the fetal to placenta ratio in spite of a decrease in birthweight. This increase is analogous to that seen at high altitude where there is a decrease in oxygen tension.

Naeye [31] confirmed the enlargement of smokers' placentas and found microscopic lesions in the placenta characteristic of underperfusion from the uterus that increase with increased smoking. Additional evidence that hypoxia is related to smoking's effect is given by the fact that it is associated with increased hemoglobin and red cell number in the cord blood [38].

Carbon monoxide does not appear to be the sole cause of smoking's effect on the fetus, for rats exposed to smoke from lettuce leaf, lettuce leaf plus nicotine, and tobacco leaf showed decreased birthweights of 9%, 12%, and 17%, respectively [10]. Thus, in addition to carbon monoxide, nicotine appears involved in smoking's effect on the fetus. Nicotine in concentrations present in the blood of smokers acts to produce vasoconstriction, and this effect on the uterine vessels might decrease placental blood flow and hence oxygenization of the fetus. In experimental studies on rhesus monkeys [37] nicotine was injected into pregnant monkeys in a concentration similar to smokers' blood nicotine levels, and decreased fetal oxygenization was documented. Decreased intervillous blood flow in response to smoking a standard cigarette has been shown for man [39]. This change in flow normalized within 15 minutes, suggesting a vasospastic response to some component in tobacco smoke, the most likely candidate being nicotine.

The third known component of tobacco smoke which may be involved in smoking's effect on the fetus and birthweight is cyanide. Subclinical cyanide poisoning may be part of the way tobacco smoke exerts its adverse effects. Cyanide may be detoxified to thiocyanate, and increased levels of thiocyanate have been documented in cord blood of infants of smoking mothers [37]. Cyanide is also detoxified by a mechanism involving vitamin B_{12}, and serum B_{12} has been shown to be lower in women who smoke [40]. Furthermore, mean B_{12} levels are lower in mothers with small babies and, therefore, the decrease in B_{12} brought about by smoking may be involved in the decreased birthweight of infants of smokers.

PREGNANCY WASTAGE

The next major question concerning smoking and pregnancy is its effect on pregnancy wastage. Spontaneous abortion rates, maternal complication rates, prematurity rates, teratology, and perinatal and neonatal morbidity and mortality have all been investigated in pregnancy.

Smoking appears to be associated with an increased rate of spontaneous abortion [9,41]. Furthermore, in studies of spontaneous abortions, smoking was associated with an increased percentage of normal karyotypes [41–43], which suggests that smoking causes its increase in spontaneous abortion rate through loss of genetically normal fetuses. The effect appears to be due to carbon monoxide-induced decidual necrosis mediated by smoking. The decidua is most sensitive to this effect at around mid-trimester [44]. Teratogenic action by smoking on the fetus does not appear to be involved, for only two studies documented a teratogenic effect. In the first study [9], based on data from the 1958 British Perinatal Mortality Study, there was a 50% increase in congenital heart disease in infants of smokers, and the teratogenicity was thus not related to spontaneous abortion. The second study showed a significant increase in the incidence of anencephaly in white smoking mothers who smoked more than ten cigarettes per day [45]. This increase in anencephaly was associated with an increased perinatal mortality but not an increased abortion rate.

The next facet of smoking's effect on pregnancy wastage is its influence on the rate of prematurity and associated perinatal mortality. Many have confirmed that smoking is associated with an increased incidence of prematurity, whether the older criterion of birthweight less than 2,500 grams [7,25,27,28] or the newer one of gestational age [2,41] is used. Naeye [31] found that in smokers the length of gestation was a mean of 1.5 days shorter than the length of gestation of nonsmokers. An increase in perinatal mortality has been documented in mothers who smoke during pregnancy in several studies [7,8,11,15,18,36,46,47]. Other studies showed a dose-response relationship with increasing perinatal mortality with increasing smoking [7,18,36,47] (Table II). This increased perinatal mortality was correlated with prematurity [7,36]. However, one study [11] showed that smokers who had low-birthweight babies had infants of higher mean birthweight and lower perinatal mortality than low-birthweight infants of controls. A change in maternal smoking at the fourth month was shown to place the patient at risk for adverse effects on the pregnancy or fetus compatible with her new smoking status [15]. The increased perinatal mortality was shown to be worse in the poor and blacks [46]; however, it was present regardless of maternal height, weight, hospital status, age-parity-group, birth place, previous pregnancy history, weight gain, time of gestation, and sex of child [18].

In addition to perinatal mortality, maternal complications associated with perinatal morbidity and mortality are increased in smokers (Table III). There is a significant increase in the incidence of placenta previa, abruptio placenta, bleeding

TABLE II. Increase in Perinatal Mortality

Source		Increase (%)
Fielding [4]	<1 PPD[a]	20
Mausner [5]	≥1 PPD	33
Mausner [5]		34.4
Butler et al [12]		28
Meyer et al [15]	<1 PPD	20
	>1 PPD	35
Rush and Kass [37]		33.4

[a]PPD = packs per day.

TABLE III. Increase in Perinatal Complications

Source		Placenta previa (%)	Abruptio placenta (%)
Fielding [4]	<1 PPD[a]	25	24
	>1 PPD	92	68
Meyer et al [15]	<1 PPD	25	23
	>1 PPD	92	86

[a]PPD = packs per day.

during pregnancy, and prolonged rupture of membranes, and these increases reflect directly the level of maternal smoking [7,18,36]. There was also an association noted between smoking and an increased incidence of amniotic fluid infection [31].

Because the highest risk of intrauterine and neonatal death in infants of smoking mothers is at 20–28 weeks [7] and, as in cases of abruptio placenta, because there is an association between decidual necrosis and smoking that is most prominent at mid-trimester [44], it is postulated that increases in maternal complications, which are mostly associated with bleeding, are due to toxic effects of smoking on the decidua. An alternate hypothesis is that they are due to carbon monoxide toxicity on the uterine arteries [36]. This thesis is supported by study of the umbilical veins of placenta from heavy smokers, which show severe changes in the intima and media similar to vessel changes observed in animal studies involving exposure to carbon monoxide, hypoxia, or nicotine [48].

LONG-TERM EFFECT ON THE CHILD

Smoking exposure in utero may have a long-term effect on both physical health and mental function of the offspring. Infants of smokers, as noted above, show decreased birthweight, and in one study [12] they showed decreased height at one year. This difference was no longer apparent at four and seven years. A second study [49] showed a decrease in weight gain and growth in length/weight at one and four years when smokers' offspring were compared to nonsmokers' offspring, and the smokers' offspring were significantly lighter in actual weight at 6½ years.

Postneonatal mortality and morbidity up to the age of five are increased in infants of smokers [11], and the incidence of bronchitis and pneumonia is more common during the first year of life in children of parents who smoke [2,50]. There is no apparent difference in the incidence of cancer in individuals exposed to tobacco smoke in utero [51]. However, there is a significant association with smoking by the mother during pregnancy and the occurrence of sudden infant death syndrome [52,53].

Infants of mothers who smoke more than 20–30 cigarettes per day and breast feed experience more gastrointestinal symptoms than controls, a finding that may be related to the decreased milk yield noted in these mothers [54], which is due to the nicotine in tobacco smoke which appears to impair milk production by its effect on prolactin release [55]. It is also possible that these infants experience some morbidity from the nicotine in their mother's breast milk, as there is a direct dose-response relationship between the amount smoked and the level of nicotine in breast milk [2].

The most disturbing deleterious long-term effect on the child may be decreased mental function and possible lowered IQ correlated with maternal smoking during pregnancy [27]. Infants of smoking mothers show delayed onset of crying [10], and in an animal study [35] rats were exposed during gestation to carbon monoxide in levels that produced carboxyhemoglobin levels equivalent to that of smokers' and their offspring showed decreased behavioral activity through the preweaning period, altered central catecholamine activity, and decreased total brain protein at birth. That total brain cell number is decreased in rats exposed to smoke during gestation has been established [16,27], and the possibility that smoking exposure prenatally may produce a permanent detrimental effect on mental function must be entertained. In an analysis of data from follow-up of the 1958 British Perinatal Mortality Study a slight retardation in reading skills at age seven in the offspring of smokers was noted [9]. Finally, hyperkinesis in children may be linked in some instances with maternal smoking, for Denson [56] showed that mothers of hyperkinetic children reported smoking two to three times as many cigarettes during pregnancy as did controls.

CONCLUSIONS

Smoking in pregnancy seems to exert many deleterious effects on the outcome of the pregnancy exposed. The major effects that have been established are 1) decreased birthweight, 2) increased spontaneous abortion rate, 3) increased perinatal mortality rate, 4) increased incidence of abruptio placenta and placenta previa, and 5) possible decreased mental function in the surviving offspring. It appears that these effects are produced through intrauterine oxygen deprivation and that the cigarette products, carbon monoxide, nicotine, and cyanide, are involved in their genesis. Because of its deleterious action, cigarette smoking should be strongly discouraged prior to pregnancy, and as there appears to be some evidence that early discontinuation of smoking in pregnancy may reduce the fetus's chance of being affected even if there has been smoking early in the first trimester, discontinuation of smoking should be stressed at the first prenatal visit.

REFERENCES

1. Sontag LT, Wallace RF: The effect of cigarette smoking during pregnancy upon the fetal heart rate. Am J Obstet Gynecol 29:77–83, 1935.
2. Highlights of the surgeon general's report on smoking and health. Morbidity and Mortality Weekly Report 28:1–11, 1979.
3. Ory HW: Association between oral contraceptives and myocardial infarction. JAMA 237: 2619–2622, 1977.
4. Jick H, Porter J, Morrison AS: Relation between smoking and age of natural menopause. Report from the Boston collaborative drug surveillance program, Boston University Medical Center. Lancet 1:1354–1355, 1977.
5. Williams RR, Horm JW: Association of cancer sites with tobacco and alcohol consumption and socioeconomic status of patients: Interview study from the third national cancer survey. J Natl Cancer Inst 58:525–547, 1977.
6. Pirani BB, Macgillivray I: Smoking during pregnancy: Its effect on maternal metabolism and fetoplacental function. Obstet Gynecol 52:257–263, 1978.
7. Fielding JE: Smoking and pregnancy. N Engl J Med 298:337–339, 1978.
8. Mausner JS: Smoking and pregnancy. Ann Intern Med 79:272, 1973.
9. Fedrick J: Possible teratogenic effect of cigarette smoking. Nature 231:529–530, 1971.
10. Longo LD: Carbon monoxide in the pregnant mother and fetus and its exchange across the placenta. Ann NY Acad Sci 174:312–341, 1970.
11. Rantakallia P: The effect of maternal smoking on birth weight and the subsequent health of the child. Early Hum Dev 2:371–382, 1978.
12. Hardy JD, Mellits ED: Does maternal smoking during pregnancy have a long-term effect on the child. Lancet 2:1332–1336, 1972.
13. Bailey RR: The effect of maternal smoking on the infant birth weight. NZ Med J 71: 293–294, 1970.
14. Miller HC, Hassancin K: Fetal malnutrition in white newborn infants, maternal factors. Pediatrics 52:504–512, 1973.
15. Butler NR, Goldstein H, Ross EM: Cigarette smoking in pregnancy: Its influence on birth weight and perinatal mortality. Br Med J 2:127–130, 1972.
16. Haworth JC: Cigarette smoking during pregnancy and the effect on the fetus. Can J Public Health 64 (Suppl):20–24, 1973.
17. Pirani BBK: Smoking during pregnancy. Obstet Gynecol Surv 33:1–13, 1978.
18. Meyer MB, Jonas BS, Tonascia JA: Perinatal events associated with maternal smoking during pregnancy. Am J Epidemiol 103:464–476, 1976.
19. Beal VA: Nutritional studies during pregnancy, II. Dietary intake, maternal weight gain, and size of infant. J Am Diet Assoc 58:321–326, 1971.
20. Cope I, Lancaster P, Stevens L: Smoking in pregnancy. Med J Aust 1:673, 1973.
21. Yerushalmy J: Mothers' cigarette smoking and survival of infants. Am J Obstet Gynecol 88:505, 1964.
22. Ravenholt RL, Levinski MJ, Nellist DJ, Takenaga M: Effects of smoking upon reproduction. Am J Obstet Gynecol 96:267–281, 1966.
23. Hickey RJ, Clelland RC, Bowers EJ: Maternal smoking, birth weight, infant death, and the self-selection problem. Am J Obstet Gynecol 131:805–811, 1978.
24. Silverman DT: Maternal smoking and birth weight. Am J Epidemiol 105:513–521, 1977.
25. Rush D: Examination of the relationship between birth weight, cigarette smoking during pregnancy and maternal weight gain. J Obstet Gynecol Br Commonw 81:746, 1974.

26. Meyer MB: How does maternal smoking affect birth weight and maternal weight gain? Evidence from the Ontario Perinatal Mortality Study. Am J Obstet Gynecol 131:888–893, 1978.
27. Longo LD: The biological effects of carbonmonoxide on the pregnant woman, fetus and newborn infant. Am J Obstet Gynecol 129:69–103, 1977.
28. McDonald RL, Lanford CF: Effects of smoking on selected clinical obstetric factors. Obstet Gynecol 26:470–475, 1965.
29. Butler NR, Goldstein H: Smoking in pregnancy and subsequent child development. Br Med J 4:573–575, 1973.
30. Buncher CR: Cigarette smoking and duration of pregnancy. Am J Obstet Gynecol 103: 942–946, 1969.
31. Naeye RL: Effects of maternal cigarette smoking on the fetus and placenta. Br J Obstet Gynecol 85:732–737, 1978.
32. Cole PV, Hawkins LH, Roberts D: Smoking during pregnancy and its effects on the fetus. J Obstet Gynecol Br Commonw 79:782–787, 1972.
33. Longo LD: Carbonmonoxide: Effects on oxygenation of the fetus in utero. Science 194: 523–525, 1976.
34. Dow TG, Rooney PJ, Spence M: Does anemia increase the risks to the fetus caused by smoking in pregnancy? Br Med J 4:253–254, 1975.
35. Fechter LD, Annau Z: Toxicity of mild prenatal carbonmonoxide exposure. Science 197: 680–682, 1977.
36. Meyer MD, Tonascia JA: Maternal smoking, pregnancy complications, and perinatal mortality. Am J Obstet Gynecol 128:494–502, 1977.
37. Editorial: Cigarette smoking in pregnancy. Br Med J 2:492–493, 1976.
38. D'Souza SW, Black PM, Williams N, Jennison RF: Effect of smoking upon the haematological values of cord blood. Br J Obstet Gynecol 85:495–499, 1978.
39. Lehtovirta P, Forss M: The acute affect of smoking on intervillous blood flow of the placenta. Br J Obstet Gynecol 85:729–731, 1978.
40. McGarry JM, Andrews J: Smoking in pregnancy and vitamin B_{12} metabolism. Br Med J 2:74–77, 1972.
41. Kline J, Stein ZA, Susser M, Warburten D: Smoking: A risk factor for spontaneous abortion. N Engl J Med 297:793–796, 1977.
42. Boue J, Bou A, Lazar P: Retrospective and prospective epidemiological studies of 1500 karyotyped spontaneous human abortions. Teratology 12:11–26, 1975.
43. Alberman E, Creasy M, Elliot M, Spicer C: Maternal factors associated with fetal chromosomal anomalies in spontaneous abortions. Br J Obstet Gynecol 83:621–627, 1976.
44. Naeye RL, Harkness WL, Utts J: Abruptio placentae and perinatal death: A prospective study. Am J Obstet Gynecol 128:740–746, 1977.
45. Naeye RL: Relationship of cigarette smoking to congenital anomalies and perinatal death. Am J Pathol 90:289–294, 1978.
46. Rush D, Kass EH: Maternal smoking: A reassessment of the association with perinatal mortality. Am J Epidemiol 96:183–196, 1972.
47. Meyer MB, Tonascia JA, Buck C: The interrelationship of maternal smoking and increased perinatal mortality with other risk factors. Further analysis of the Ontario Perinatal Mortality Study, 1960–1961. Am J Epidemiol 100:443–452, 1974.
48. Asmussen I: Ultrastructure of human umbilical veins, observations on veins from newborn children of smoking and nonsmoking mothers. Acta Obstet Gynecol Scand 47:253–255, 1978.

49. Dunn HG, McGurney A, Ingram S, Hunter CM: Maternal cigarette smoking and the child's subsequent development: I. Physical growth to the age of 6½ years. Can J Public Health 67:499–505, 1976.
50. Colley JRT, Holland WW, Corkhill RT: Influence of passive smoking and parental phlegm pneumonia and bronchitis in early childhood. Lancet 2:1031–1034, 1974.
51. Neutel CI, Buck C: Effect of smoking during pregnancy on the risk of cancer in children. J Natl Cancer Inst 47:59–63, 1971.
52. Bergman AB, Wiesner LA: Relationship of passive cigarette smoking to sudden infant death syndrome Pediatrics 58:665–668, 1976.
53. Naeye RL, Ladis B, Drage JS: Sudden infant death syndrome. Am J Dis Child 180: 1207–1210, 1976.
54. Forrest JM: Drugs in pregnancy and lactation. Med J Aust 2:138–141, 1976.
55. Blake CA, Sawyer CH: Nicotine blocks the suckling induced rise in circulating prolactin in lactating rats. Science 177:619–621, 1972.
56. Denson R, Nanson JJ, Mcwatters MA: Hyperkinesis and maternal smoking. Can Psychiatr Assoc J 20:183–187, 1975.

Neurobehavioral Effects of Prenatal Origin: Sex Hormones

Heino F. L. Meyer-Bahlburg, Dr Rer Nat, and Anke A. Ehrhardt, PhD

The use of sex hormones in the treatment of problem pregnancies was first introduced in the 1940s after it had become known that successful initiation as well as maintenance of pregnancy depended to a large extent on hormones produced by the mother as well as by the feto-placental unit. High-risk pregnancies such as those threatened by spontaneous abortion, premature birth, stillbirth, or congenital abnormalities, often in conjunction with pathologic states of the pregnant mother, such as diabetes or toxemia of pregnancy, were linked to deficiencies of hormone production, and supplementation seemed to be the logical approach to treatment. Since most steroid hormones have some progestational properties, a great variety of hormone preparations were tried, expecially progestogens and estrogens. Some of the hormones used were soon discarded because of unwanted side-effects. This was particularly true of the androgenic hormones, which had virilizing effects on the mother and masculinizing effects on the genitals of genetic female offspring. Such androgenic effects were also found in certain progestogens that had been derived from androgenic hormones but that were structurally quite different. More recently, even more severe and potentially lethal side-effects have become known to occur with a widely used nonsteroidal estrogen, diethylstilbestrol (DES); when administered during pregnancy, this drug causes minor genital abnormalities in a large number of both male and female offspring and a rare type of vaginal cancer (clear cell adenocarcinoma) in a small but significant number of female offspring.

An additional source of exposure to exogenous hormones during pregnancy is the widespread use of hormonal oral contraceptives, which are often inadvertently taken during the initial stages of pregnancy before the mother is aware that she has conceived.

Modified and updated version of a paper by the authors published in: Youngs DD and Ehrhardt AA (eds), Psychosomatic Obstetrics and Gynecology, New York: Appleton Century Crofts, 1979, pp 3–17.

Drug and Chemical Risks to the Fetus and Newborn:93–107
Published 1980 Alan R. Liss, Inc., 150 Fifth Avenue, New York, NY 10011

Two lines of thought led us to expect that hormone treatment of problem pregnancies might well have effects on the developing nervous system of the fetus, and, thereby, on later behavior. First, it is well known that problem pregnancies predispose the surviving offspring to neurological and intellectual deficits. Any treatment that effectively diminishes the pregnancy risk can be expected to also decrease the rate of such fetal abnormalities. A second source of evidence for behavioral effects of hormones is animal research, which has conclusively demonstrated that there is a sensitive period of the development of the hypothalamus and adjacent structures of the brain during which sex hormones have a major function in the differentiation of sex-dimorphic systems that regulate gonadotropin secretion and or behavior. Thus, it would seem mandatory to screen hormones used to improve "at-risk" pregnancies for behavioral effects and not to limit the study of their effectiveness to rates of spontaneous abortion, premature birth, infant mortality and morbidity, and the evaluation of their side-effects to the well-being of the mother and to congenital malformations of the newborn. The required behavioral studies need to involve long-term follow-up and pose tremendous logistical problems. Because of this, only a handful of pertinent studies is available, most of them afflicted by serious methodological inadequacies. The crucial methodological question is usually the selection of controls, which must not only be comparable in age and sex but in less obvious characteristics such as pregnancy history, socioeconomic level, and social factors that led to comparable chances for medical treatment in the case of a problem pregnancy.

EFFECTS ON PSYCHOSEXUAL DIFFERENTIATION

Introduction

The term "psychosexual differentiation" refers to the development of gender identity – ie, the primary identification with the female or male sex – and of sex-dimorphic behavior, which encompasses all those aspects of behavior in which normal girls and boys differ from each other in our culture and at this time in history. Extensive animal research has shown that some of the major aspects of sex-dimorphic behavior, such as mating behavior, parenting, and aggression, are to quite an extent dependent on the effects of sex hormones during a critical period of brain development early in prenatal or perinatal development. If the fetus, regardless of genetic sex, is exposed to androgens during this critical period (and has appropriate hormone receptors available), its hypothalamus and adjacent areas of the brain will be organized so as to facilitate the expression of male behavior later in life, especially under the influence of pubertal hormones. Conversely, when androgens are absent or the fetus lacks appropriate receptors – ie, the brain is unresponsive to male sex hormones – brain differentiation will be along female lines [Money and Ehrhardt, 1972]. This is the classical organization hypothesis of sex-dimorphic behavior. Recent revisions of this theory [Goy and Goldfoot,

1975] include hormones other than androgens. Progesterone, for instance, is recognized as a hormone that counteracts androgens and, thereby, may protect the brain of female fetuses in certain species from the effects of available androgens. Moreover, current theories consider that androgens may have to be converted into estrogens on the target cell level in order to exert their decisive effects on target cell nuclei; this hypothesis would explain why pharmacologic doses of exogenous estrogens may, in fact, have masculinizing effects in females of various species.

Although nobody doubts that social learning plays a much greater role in human behavior than in subhuman mammals, there is sufficient evidence to suggest that biological factors influence psychosexual differentiation in man, too. Anatomically and histologically, the subcortical regions of the human brain have a striking similarity to those of subhuman mammals. The timing of peak androgen production by the fetal testes corresponds closely to the timing of hypothalamic differentiation as it does in the prenatal or perinatal lower mammal. And, finally, there are syndromes of prenatal endocrine abnormalities, such as congenital virilizing adrenal hyperplasia in the female and androgen insensitivity in the genetic male, which provide interesting models for the effects of prenatal androgens or of their deficiency on human sex-dimorphic behavior. Various studies have been reported on samples of patients suffering from such syndromes; the overall conclusion is that gender identity follows closely the sex of assignment and rearing, whereas sex-dimorphic behavior, regardless of the genetic sex of the individual, shows marked influences of prenatal hormones in the expected direction, although the sex-dimorphic behaviors usually stay within the general range of accepted behavior for the specific gender [Money and Ehrhardt, 1972; Ehrhardt, 1975]. If psychosocial development in humans is influenced by prenatal endocrine abnormalities, the question arises whether prenatal hormone treatment will have analogous effects also. If so, then androgenic steroids should produce some masculinization of behavior; progesterone and related compounds would be expected to counteract androgenic effects; and estrogens either might have masculinizing effects or demasculinizing effects, depending on the kind of hormone and its dosage. Behavioral follow-up studies of offspring from hormone-treated pregnancies have so far been restricted to treatment regimens involving progestogens or progestogen–estrogen combinations.

Progestogens

Subsumed under the category "progestogens" are both naturally occurring and synthetic progestational agents that are chemically closely related to either progesterone or to androgenic steroids, in spite of their much reduced androgenic action. Masculinization of female fetuses has been found after treatment with either class of hormones. However, only very rare individual cases of masculinization after prenatal exposure to exogenous progesterone [eg, Wilkins, 1960] or to derivatives such as medroxyprogesterone acetate (MPA) [eg, Burstein et al, 1964] have been reported, and a causal relationship has not been established beyond doubt. Almost equally rare are reports suggesting antiandrogenic effects of the same exogenous progestogens, based on the observation in a few human newborn males of an association of hypospadias with progestogen treatment during pregnancy [eg, Aarskog, 1971]. On the other hand, a significant minority of female fetuses exposed to androgen-derived progestogens has shown genital masculinization frequently enough that a causal relationship is generally assumed, although the mechanism of action is not yet understood. It is important to note that the overwhelming majority of newborns from progestogen-treated pregnancies shows normal external genitalia. The evidence for this statement comes from such studies as the national Collaborative Perinatal Project, which investigated 1,144 mother–child pairs who had been exposed to progestogens as progestational agents or contraceptives during the first four months of pregnancy: only 13 of these children – compared to an expected number of 11.1 for offspring not exposed to these drugs – showed any disorders of the genitourinary system, including hypospadias; the trivial difference is not statistically significant [Heinonen et al, 1977]. Such findings, however, do not rule out a higher prevalence rate of hormonal CNS effects since the utilization of hormones in the periphery is known to be mediated through different biochemical pathways than (at least parts of) the utilization of hormones by brain tissues.

The only psychological study of a sample of girls with prenatal masculinization due to androgen-derived progestogens was described by Ehrhardt and Money. They published a preliminary report, without control groups, on psychosexual development in 1967. Later reports [Ehrhardt, 1969; Money and Ehrhardt, 1972] included comparisons with pair-matched controls involving detailed blind rating procedures. The hormone-treated sample consisted of ten girls, aged three to 14 years, at the time of study, nine of whom were born with somewhat masculinized external genitalia (which was the reason for their selection for this study) and surgically feminized if necessary; the tenth was the unmasculinized but also hormone-treated sibling of one of the subjects. The detailed behavioral interviews with the subjects and their mothers brought interesting results. Nine index subjects were rated to be tomboys; progestogen treatment was associated with increased athletic interests and skills, preference for male versus female playmates, for utilitarian and functional rather than traditionally feminine clothing, for toy cars, guns, etc, versus dolls, and a priority of career over marriage. In spite of the long-term tomboyism exhibited by these girls, their gender identity was feminine. There is also no evidence that such girls, after puberty, develop a homosexual orientation [Mathews and Money, 1978]. The mothers of patients and controls did not differ systematically in their reports of child rearing practices [Ehrhardt, 1969]. Thus, it seems that along with the masculinizing effect on the genitalia, these androgen-derived hormones also have masculinizing effects on the brain, which is in good agreement with the findings on girls with congenital virilizing adrenal hyperplasia

[Ehrhardt, 1978], who also show behavioral effects of prenatal masculinization.

More widespread than the use of androgen-derived progestogens has been treatment with progesterone-related progestogens. It is for these types of progestogens that Dorfman and Kincl [1963] originally suggested that progesterone may protect the developing hypothalamic–pituitary–gonadal system of the fetus against possibly damaging effects of increases in androgen (and/or estrogen) concentrations. Later findings of sex differences in fetal and/or neonatal progesterone levels in the rhesus monkey and the rat – with the females having the higher levels – led to general models of an interaction of progesterone with other sex steroids in both male and female fetuses [Resko, 1974; Shapiro et al, 1976]. According to this theory, progesterone protects the female brain from the masculinizing effects of androgens and estrogens. There are only three studies that concern such effects in humans. Zussman et al [1975, 1977] examined 12 females and 18 males, age 16–19 years, who had been exposed in utero to exogenous progesterone, which was administered for the relief of precursor symptoms of pre-eclamptic toxemia. In a blind interview study, the hormone-exposed subjects were compared to 29 matched controls, six of whom were offspring from untreated toxemic pregnancies. Progesterone exposure in boys correlated negatively with physical activity level in childhood and also with heterosexual activity level in adolescence. In girls, progesterone exposure was negatively correlated with reports of tomboyism and positively with traditionally feminine activities in childhood. Effects on gender identity were not reported. The data on sex-dimorphic behaviors are compatible with the hypothesized anti-androgenic action of progesterone. Unfortunately, the preliminary reports by Zussman et al give insufficient information on the subjects' background variables, so that one cannot decide whether the behavioral differences described are really due to the progesterone treatment itself and not to differences in pregnancy conditions or socioeconomic level.

Lynch, Mychalkiw and Hutt [1978] studied another sample of female and male adolescents (age 16 years) with a history of prenatal progesterone exposure, in this case administered for the prevention of pre-eclamptic toxemia. Nineteen experimental subjects and thirteen controls were compared with regard to two personality questionnaires, the Eysenck Personality Inventory (EPI) and a modified Mf (masculinity-femininity) sub-scale of the MMPI. There was only one significant difference between hormone treated subjects and controls: the progesterone exposed females (N = 13) scored significantly lower than the control females (N = 7) on the EPI sub-scale Extraversion. Extraversion, however, does not represent one of the typically sex-dimorphic behaviors and the composition of the female experimental and control samples does not permit to ascribe the test score difference unambiguously to a progesterone effect.

The behavioral sequelae of medroxyprogesterone acetate (MPA) were investigated in a double-blind interview study by Meyer-Bahlburg and Ehrhardt. The study samples were selected from the Buffalo branch of the Collaborative Perinatal Project, in which approximately 2,400 children were followed from the early months of pregnancy to age seven years, with frequent medical and psychometric examinations. Thirteen boys [Meyer-Bahlburg et al, 1977] and 15 girls [Ehrhardt et al, 1977] who were exposed to MPA exclusively and to no other exogenous hormone underwent a double-blind interview study together with control subjects from the same population with documented absence of prenatal hormone treatment who were very closely pairwise matched for sex, race, birth date, and socioeconomic level, and as much as possible for vaginal bleeding during pregnancy (there were no diabetic pregnancies in the sample, and only very few cases with (mild) symptoms of toxemia, at the end of pregnancy). Systematic half-structured interviews were conducted with both mother and child separately. Systematic ratings were done by two independent raters. No behavioral differences were found between hormone-exposed males (aged eight to 14 years) and controls, and even no consistent behavioral trends. Significantly fewer hormone-exposed girls than controls were being leveled a tomboy during childhood, and more of them showed a consistent preference for feminine clothing styles. Nonsignificant trends for other variables went in the same direction. Gender identity seemed not to be affected but was unambiguously female in all subjects. Again, the results on sex-dimorphic behavior are compatible with the theory of an antiandrogenic action of prenatal progesterone. That the MPA study showed hormone effects in the girls, but not in the boys, might be due to the lower dosage of progestogen administered to the mothers of this study, in comparison to the dosage used on the mothers in the sample of Zussman and coworkers [Ehrhardt et al, 1977].

In summary, the four studies available on the effects of prenatal progestogen on sex-dimorphic behavior seem to support the theory of hormone-influenced differentiation of sex-dimorphic behavior in man; androgen-derived progestogens seem to have shifted the behavior of girls to the masculine side, whereas progesterone and MPA show opposite effects. It is important to note, however, that the effects observed in both the progesterone and MPA studies were weak, even with relatively high-dosage treatment, as in the London sample described by Zussman et al [1975, 1977], and it seems possible that the effects have been brought about by factors other than hormones, for instance by pregnancy conditions. Further doubts about the validity of the progesterone theory are raised by recent data that fail to establish any sex difference in progesterone levels of umbilical cord blood at term [Tulchinsky and Okada, 1975; Dawood and Helmkamp, 1977]. In this respect, humans seem to differ from lower mammals. Thus, we can say that there is some weak corroborative evidence for the theory that progesterone has an androgen-protective effect on the developing brain but that the theory cannot be considered confirmed for the human situation.

Progestogen-Estrogen Combinations

In subhuman mammals, exogenous estrogens administered prenatally or perinatally exert seemingly paradoxical effects on genital morphology and sex-dimorphic behavior; that is, they tend to masculinize females and to demasculinize males. Analogous paradoxical modifications of the genitalia have been found in a few scattered cases of human infants after exposure to the nonsteroidal estrogen, diethylstilbestrol (DES) [summarized in Bongiovanni, 1976] ; the rarity of such cases, however, precludes stringent causal inferences. Estrogen is rarely used alone for the treatment of problem pregnancies, and behavioral studies of offspring from pregnancies treated solely with estrogens are not yet available. The more common treatment regimen is a progestogen–estrogen combination. Since we do not have sufficient knowledge of the behavioral effects of the individual estrogens or progestogens, it is impossible to predict with any certainty their interactive effects on sex-dimorphic behavior.

If we could take for proven that prenatal progesterone has an anti-androgenic effect on the brain, and estrogen alone a masculinizing effect on females and a demasculinizing effect on males, then a simple progesterone–estrogen combination should produce demasculinization in males, while the combined effects of the two drugs on females would depend on the dosage of progesterone relative to estrogen. Such a simple hormone combination was studied by Yalom et al [1973] ; they examined a sample of twenty 16–17-year-old males who had been exposed in utero to progesterone plus DES as a medication for diabetic pregnancy. The subjects were slightly but significantly lower than untreated controls in aggression/assertion (rank order ratings on the basis of interview data sheets) and in athletic coordination (by observational ratings) and showed tendencies of overall decreased masculine interests and decreased heterosexual experience. Increased gender-identity problems or homosexuality were not noted. The same report covers another group of 20 boys at age six years who had been prenatally exposed to hydroxyprogesterone acetate in combination with estradiol valerate, again as a treatment for diabetic pregnancy; two of the index subjects had hypospadias. This group of hormone-treated boys showed decreased assertion and decreased athletic ability (by teacher ratings). Unfortunately, the control groups used in either study did not involve adequate pair-matching of children with the same intrauterine history but without hormone treatment. For instance, Yalom et al stated that the untreated diabetic mothers of control subjects had less severe forms of diabetes than the hormone-treated mothers of experimental subjects. Thus, the observed behavioral differences could be due to the medical condition of the mother as well as to the hormone treatment itself. Against a hormonal interpretation speaks also the fact that of the 16-year-old group, the subjects with the lower hormone dose and the later onset of treatment had a higher frequency of femininity ratings than high dose-late initiation subjects, and that this trend was reversed in the six-year-old group.

Hormonal effects on sex-dimorphic behavior become totally unpredictable when the study sample involves diverse combinations of a variety of estrogens and progestogens. Such a sample was studied by Reinisch and Karow [1977; and Reinisch, 1977]. They administered the Cattell Personality Questionnaires to 71 children (26 boys, 45 girls), aged five to 17 years, who had been exposed prenatally to various combinations of synthetic progestogens and estrogens, with untreated siblings as controls. In attempting to deal with the issue of hormone heterogeneity, Reinisch and Karow partitioned their sample into three groups: one group with exclusive or predominant estrogen treatment, another group with exclusive or predominant progestogen treatment, and a third group in between. The questionnaire data showed significant treatment effects: subjects who were mainly exposed to progestogens were characterized as more independent, sensitive, self-assured, individualistic, and self-sufficient, while subjects who were predominantly exposed to estrogens were more group-oriented and group-dependent. Unfortunately, this study does not permit any conclusions with regard to sex-dimorphic behavior, since the latter is not assessed by the questionnaires used and the study subjects were not analzyed by sex. The questionnaire results are hard to interpret. Although behavioral group differences might be expected on the basis of the fact that prenatal and perinatal complications were far more frequent in the hormone-exposed groups than in the sibling controls, the published reports do not allow an analysis of the three subgroups formed with regard to the different rates of prenatal complications. Even if the three subgroups did not differ with respect to complication rates (in fact, these differences were statistically controlled for by analysis of covariance) the replicability of the results would still be in doubt because of the variety of drug combinations included, the varying combinations of both sexes in all groups, and the statistical method used ($3 \times 2 \times 2$ analysis of covariance design with three covariates).

In summarizing this section, we have to say that the few studies available on the behavioral effects of prenatal progestogen—estrogen treatment in man suggest a hormonal impact, but the methodology employed does not permit us to accept the results without major reservations as to their replicability and interpretation.

EFFECTS ON INTELLECTUAL DEVELOPMENT

Introduction

The rationale for screening prenatal hormone drugs for their effects on intelligence is twofold. First, there is the well-documented fact that problem pregnancies constitute a risk for neuropsychological and intellectual deficits in the surviving offspring. This has been conclusively demonstrated, for example, for children from diabetic pregnancies, particularly when maternal diabetes is accompanied by acetonuria [Churchill et al, 1969; Stehbens et al, 1977], and for toxemia of pregnancy, especially when leading to infants who are small for gestational age [Friedman and Neff, 1977]. (Negative effects of toxemia on mental development have also been reported by Bailey [1963] and Barker and Edwards [1967].) Any treatment of such pregnancy pathologies that positively affects pregnancy outcome in terms of reduced fetal wastage, stillbirth, prematurity, and low birthweight is likely to decrease rates of neuropsychological deficit and of intellectual impairment in children from such pregnancies.

The other reason for including mental ability measures is an extension of the studies of sex-dimorphic behavior in general. Sex differences apply to strengths and weaknesses in some mental abilities; for instance, verbal ability tends to be higher in girls, and spatial perception in boys [Maccoby and Jacklin, 1974]. With appropriate tests, these differences can already be shown in elementary school age [see, for instance, Goldberg and Meredith, 1975] and may become more marked in puberty [for instance, Waber, 1976, 1977]. Inasmuch as sex differences in mental abilities are influenced by the same biological variables as other sex-dimorphic behaviors, they may be similarly affected by prenatal hormones.

Progestogens

Effects of exogenous prenatal progestogens on subsequent cognitive functioning have been studied by several teams. In their report on ten girls with prenatal progestogen treatment, mentioned earlier, Ehrhardt and Money [1967] also presented data on intelligence. None of the girls had an IQ under 100, and six were above 130. Since no control group had been used for the assessment of intelligence (the controls selected later for behavior comparisons were matched for IQ), it is not clear to what extent these unusually high IQs were a reflection of the elevated socioeconomic status of the subjects rather than an outcome of pregnancy treatment.

A series of progesterone studies was reported by Dalton [1968] in England. She examined children whose mothers had been treated with high dosages of progesterone for pre-eclamptic toxemia of pregnancy. A pilot study of 32 children, age 6–13 years, showed that the offspring of these mothers received intelligence ratings of "above average" by their head teachers slightly more frequently than the children of a matched normal control group. Dalton then investigated the offspring of mothers with toxemic pregnancies who had been random assigned to the progesterone treatment or to a non-progesterone control condition. At age one year, the 29 progesterone-exposed chidlren appeared somewhat more advanced in standing and, possibly, in walking but not with regard to other developmental milestones. Dalton also compared a sample of twenty-nine 9–10-year-old progesterone-exposed children to normal controls and to untreated toxemic controls, and teacher ratings suggested elevated school performance significantly more frequently for the hormone-exposed subjects than for both groups of controls. In a recent follow-up study of 34 progesterone-exposed children from toxemic pregnancies, Dalton [1976] reported that a higher proportion of exposed children than normal or untreated toxemic controls left school with advanced grades and entered a university. While the three samples of Dalton [1968] are independent from each other, the recently studied group seems to include subjects from the earlier samples. Unfortunately, the reports lack detail in data presentation, statistical analysis, and background information so that it is difficult to judge to what degree confounding variables have been controlled. Lynch and Mychalkiw [1978; see also Dalton, 1978 and Lynch, 1978] reanalyzed Dalton's [1968, 1976] data with statistical standard procedures and showed that almost all differences previously reported between progesterone-exposed and control groups were statistically insignificant.

Zussman et al [1975, 1977] tested a sample of 30 progesterone-exposed subjects, aged 16–19 years, which included subjects from Dalton's [1968] 9–10-year-old group and additional adolescents from Dalton's general practice, and compared them to 29 controls. These authors did not use a test of general intelligence but a number of subtests of the Differential Aptitude Test and noted elevations in several subtests, statistically significant only for Numerical Ability. Their preliminary report does not yet permit conclusive interpretations, and, as in the earlier studies by Dalton, the major problem seems to be the control group selection.

Lynch et al [1978] examined two further samples from Dalton's treatment program; here, progesterone treatment had been limited to the second and third trimester of pregnancy (starting between the 16th and 28th week). One study involved a new sample of 2-year olds, 20 of whom were progesterone treated and 13 untreated controls. They did not differ significantly in the Mental Development Index (MDI) or the Motor Development Index of the Bayley Scales of Infant Development. The second study concerned 15 progesterone-treated and 11 control subjects of Dalton's [1968] first-year sample, now 16 years old. Again, prenatal progesterone treatment was not found to be associated with elevated intelligence (Wechsler IQs) and also not with advanced academic performance as rated by teachers. However, also the results of these two studies have to be interpreted with caution because of unsatisfactory comparability of experimental and control subjects.

In their previously mentioned studies of 28 boys and girls with prenatal MPA treatment, in comparison to 28 closely pair-matched controls, Meyer-Bahlburg and Ehrhardt [1977] also investigated intelligence, using the Wechsler Intelligence Scale for Children Revised. Mean IQ for hormone-treated subjects was 108.2 and for control subjects 109.9, a statistically nonsignificant trivial difference. Although this study appears to have applied considerably stricter criteria for control-group matching, the results do not necessarily refute Dalton's data, since she used another hormone in considerably higher dosage on a differently defined sample.

However, strong arguments can be mustered against the notion that exogenous progesterone may be effective in preventing CNS damage resulting from high-risk pregnancies. Double-blind control studies of progesterone and other progestogens have failed to demonstrate improvement of outcome of high-risk pregnancies in terms of decreased rates of spontaneous abortion, prematurity, low birthweight, etc [see for instance, Fuchs & Stakemann, 1960; Øvlisen and Iversen, 1963; Shearman and Garrett, 1963; Goldzieher, 1964; Levine, 1964; Møller and Fuchs, 1965]. In fact, when Lynch and Mychalkiw [1978] reanalyzed statistically Dalton's [1962] own data from control trials of progesterone treatment in toxemia, all differences were statistically insignificant. Moreover, recent endocrine studies have shown that progesterone levels are within normal limits or even slightly elevated in such high-risk pregnancy conditions as pre-eclampsia or diabetes [see references in Vande Wiele et al, 1976]. Also, Escarcena et al [1978] have demonstrated that, at term, only about 1% of the maternally circulating progesterone crosses the placenta, making up 10% or less of the hormone in fetal circulation. If these figures apply to earlier states of pregnancies as well, even the highest treatment dosage reported (300 mg im daily [Dalton, 1968]), which is roughly equivalent to the maternal production rate of progesterone, would not contribute more than about 10% to the fetal circulation; and less extreme treatment regimens would remain far below this figure. The same arguments apply to the presumptive positive effects of progesterone on brain development in normal pregnancy. Recent attempts to replicate such progesterone effects on the rat level, in terms of neurophysiological indices and of learning behavior, have been unsuccessful or led to inconsistent results [Coyle et al, 1976; Hull et al, 1977; Snyder et al, 1979].

Data on sex-dimorphic cognitive abilities are even more scant. Zussman et al [1975, 1977] selected several subtests of the Differential Aptitude Test for the purpose of screening for hormone effects on certain sex-dimorphic abilities; they found statistically significant progesterone effects only for numerical ability and not for the typical sex-dimorphic ability subtests such as spatial reasoning. Meyer-Bahlburg and Ehrhardt [1977], in analyzing their data for the Wechsler Intelligence Scale for Children Revised, did not find any hormone-related differences in verbal or performance IQ, in Cohen's verbal, number, and Perceptual Factors, or in individual subtests. Lynch et al [1978] administered the Gottschaldt Embedded Figure Test and certain other verbal and visual tasks to their 16-year-old subjects; no progesterone effects emerged. Thus, there is no evidence in any of the three studies that prenatal hormone influences sex-dimorphic cognitive abilities.

Progestogen-Estrogen Combinations

The reasoning underlying the follow-up studies of intellectual development after prenatal progestogen treatment also applies to progestogen–estrogen combinations. To date, relevant data have been published only by Reinisch and Karow [1977] on the same sample as described above. The average Full IQ for all treated subjects was 121.85 as compared to the untreated siblings' mean score of 119.92; the difference is far from statistically significant. Breaking the total group up into the three subgroups described before did not influence the results. Also, the addition of covariates did not alter them. The authors did not do specific analyses for sex-dimorphic cognitive abilities.

With regard to the latter, there is only one isolated finding: Yalom et al [1973], in their previously described study on diabetic pregnancies, found that the experimental group performed significantly poorer on the sex-dimorphic Embedded Figure Test, a test of field dependence–independence in perception in which females perform poorer on average than males, than normal controls and diabetic controls. Due to questions of sample comparability as discussed before, it is not clear if this result can be ascribed to the hormone treatment or the pregnancy condition.

CONCLUSIONS

Sex-Dimorphic Behavior

Data from the few available studies on the effects of prenatal progestogens on sex-dimorphic behavior are compatible with the animal research based theory regarding the role of prenatal hormone influences in psychosexual differentiation. The empirical evidence suggests masculinizing brain effects of androgen-derived progestogens, anti-androgen effects of progesterone and related compounds and of progestogen-estrogen combinations, the latter in males only. Best established is the role of prenatal androgen-derived progestogens, especially when seen in conjunction with previous studies on patients with hyperandrogenizing endocrine conditions. The evidence for an anti-androgenic action of prenatal progesterone and related compounds seems insufficient as yet and open to different interpretations. No effect of prenatal exogenous hormones was shown on the development of gender identity in the three studies that included this aspect of psychosexual differentiation [Ehrhardt and Money, 1967; Meyer-Bahlburg et al, 1977; Ehrhardt et al, 1977]. Generally, the data are not strong enough to constitute a genuine confirmation of the psychoendocrine theory of psychosexual differentiation. However, in spite of the methodological deficiencies of the studies reviewed, the evidence is too suggestive to be discarded without more decisive contrary empirical evidence. It is of clinical importance that none of the behavioral studies reviewed here has shown any noteworthy psychopathologic side-effects of progestogen and estrogen treatment during pregnancy on the offspring.

Intelligence

The results of studies on the effects of prenatal sex hormones on general intelligence are fairly negative. Especially the relatively well-controlled studies seem to indicate a lack of any positive effects, which is in agreement with the current state of our knowledge of the largely unimportant role of progestogens and estrogens in the etiology and treatment of the more common abnormal pregnancy conditions. In particular, hormone treatment for the purpose of elevating the offspring's IQ seems unwarranted. Effects of prenatal sex hormones on sex-dimorphic cognitive abilities have not been found in the three studies that investigated this issue.

ACKNOWLEDGMENTS

This work was supported in part by a grant from the Spencer Foundation.

REFERENCES

Aarskog D: Intersex conditions masquerading as simple hypospadias. In Bergsma D (ed): "The Endocrine System," Part X. Baltimore: Williams & Wilkins for the National Foundation–March of Dimes. BD: OAS VII (6):122–130, 1971.

Bailey MA: Toxemia of pregnancy: Cognitive and emotional effects in children from consistent and non-consistent environments. PhD thesis. Ann Arbor, Michigan: Xerox University Microfilms, 1963.

Barker DJP, Edwards JH: Obstetric complications and school performance. Br Med J 3:695–699, 1967.

Bongiovanni AM: Androgens, estrogens, and the fetus. In New MI, Fiser RH Jr (eds): "Diabetes and Other Endocrine Disorders During Pregnancy and in the Newborn." New York: Alan R Liss, Inc, 1976, pp 173–178.

Burstein R, Wasserman HC: The effect of provera on the fetus. Obstet Gynecol 23:931–934, 1964.

Churchill JA, Berendes HW, Nemore J: Neuropsychological deficits in children of diabetic mothers. Am J Obstet Gynecol 105:257–268, 1969.

Coyle IR, Anker R, Cragg B: Behavioral, biochemical and histological effects of prenatal administration of progesterone in the rat. Pharmacol Biochem Behav 5:587–590, 1976.

Dalton K: Controlled trials in the prophylactic value of progesterone in the treatment of pre-eclamptic toxaemia. J Obstet Gynaec Br Commonw 69:463–468, 1962.

Dalton K: Ante-natal progesterone and intelligence. Br J Psychiatry 114:1377–1382, 1968.

Dalton K: Prenatal progesterone and educational attainments. Br J Psychiatry 129:438–442, 1976.

Dalton K: Prenatal progesterone. (Letter to the Editor). Early Hum Dev 2:393–394, 1978.

Dawood MY, Helmkamp F: Human umbilical arterial and venous progesterone concentrations. Obstet Gynecol 50:450–453, 1977.

Dorfman RM, Kincl FA: A new function of progesterone. IV. Reunion Anual, Soc. Mexicana Nutricion y Endocrinologia, December, p 171, 1963. (Cited in Dorfman RI: The anti-

estrogenic and antiandrogenic activities of progesterone in the defense of a normal fetus. Anat Rec 157:547–558, 1967).
Ehrhardt AA: Zur Wirkung fötaler Hormone auf Intelligenz und geschlechtsspezifisches Verhalten. PhD thesis, University of Düsseldorf, Düsseldorf, 1969 (in German).
Ehrhardt AA: Prenatal hormone exposure and psychosexual differentiation. In Sachar EJ (ed): "Topics in Psychoendocrinology. New York: Grune & Stratton, 1975, pp 67–82.
Ehrhardt AA: Behavioral sequelae of prenatal hormonal exposure in animals and man. In Lipton MA, DiMascio A, Killam KF (eds): "Psychopharmacology: A Generation of Progress." New York, Raven Press, 1978, pp 531–539.
Ehrhardt AA, Grisanti GC, Meyer-Bahlburg HFL: Prenatal exposure to medroxyprogesterone acetate (MPA) in girls. Psychoneuroendocrinology 2:391–398, 1977.
Ehrhardt AA, Money J: Progestin-induced hermaphroditism: IQ and psychosexual identity in a study of ten girls. J Sex Res 3:83–100, 1967.
Escarcena L, Clark H, Gurpide E: Contribution of maternal circulation to blood-borne progesterone in the fetus. I. Studies on human subjects. Am J Obstet Gynecol 130:462–465, 1978.
Friedman EA, Neff RK: Pregnancy hypertension. A systematic evaluation of clinical diagnostic criteria. Littleton, Massachusetts PSG Publishing Co., 1977.
Fuchs F, Stakemann G: Treatment of threatened premature labor with large doses of progesterone. Am J Obstet Gynecol 79:172–176, 1960.
Goldberg J, Meredith W: A longitudinal study of spatial ability. Behav Genet 5:127–135, 1975.
Goldzieher JW: Double-blind trial of a progestin in habitual abortion. JAMA 188:651–654, 1964.
Goy RW, Goldfoot DA: Neuroendocrinology: Animal models and problems of human sexuality. Arch Sex Behav 4:405–420, 1975.
Heinonen O, Slone D, Shapiro S: Birth Defects and Drugs in Pregnancy. Littleton, Massachusetts: Publishing Sciences Group, Inc, 1977.
Hull EM, Franz JR, Snyder AM: Paper presented at Annual Neurosciences Meeting, Anaheim, Calif, 1977.
Levine L: Habitual abortion. A controlled study of progestational therapy. West J Surg Obstet Gynecol 72:30–36, 1964.
Lynch A: Prenatal progesterone. (Reply): Early Hum Dev 2:394–395, 1978.
Lynch A, Mychalkiw W, Hutt SJ: Prenatal progesterone I. Its effect on development and on intellectual and academic achievement. Early Hum Dev 2:305–322, 1978.
Lynch A, Mychalkiw W: Prenatal Progesterone II. Its role in the treatment of pre-eclamptic toxaemia and its effect on the offspring's intelligence: A reappraisal. Early Hum Dev 2:323–339, 1978.
Maccoby EE, Jacklin CN: The psychology of sex differences. Stanford, California: Stanford University Press, 1974.
Mathews D, Money J: Progestin-induced hermaphroditism: A follow-up report. In Eastern Conference on Reproductive Behavior, Madison, Wisconsin, May 31–June 03, 1978. Program and Abstracts, 1978, p 62.
Meyer-Bahlburg HFL, Ehrhardt AA: Effects of prenatal hormone treatment on mental abilities. In Gemme R, Wheeler CC (eds): "Progress in Sexology." New York: Plenum Press, 1977, pp 85–92.
Meyer-Bahlburg HFL, Grisanti GC, Ehrhardt AA: Prenatal effects of sex hormones on human male behavior: Medroxyprogesterone acetate (MPA). Psychoneuroendocrinology 2:383–390, 1977.
Møller KJA, Fuchs F: Double-blind controlled trial of 6-methyl,17-acetoxyprogesterone in threatened abortion. J Obstet Gynaecol Br Commonw 72:1042–1044, 1965.

Money J, Ehrhardt AA: "Man and Woman, Boy and Girl: The Differentiation and Dimorphism of Gender Identity from Conception to Maturity." Baltimore: The Johns Hopkins University Press, 1972.

Øvlisen B, Iversen J: Treatment of threatened premature labor with 6α-methyl-17α-acetoxy-progesterone. Am J Obstet Gynecol 86:291–295, 1963.

Reinisch JM: Prenatal exposure of human fetuses to synthetic progestin and estrogen affects personality. Nature 266:561–562, 1977.

Reinisch JM, Karow WG: Prenatal exposure to synthetic progestins and estrogens: Effects on human development. Arch Sex Behav 6:257–288, 1977.

Resko JA: The relationship between fetal hormones and the differentiation of the central nervous system in primates. In Montagna W, Sadler WA (eds): "Reproductive Behavior." New York: Plenum Press, 1974, pp 211–222.

Shapiro BH, Goldman AS, Bongiovanni AM, Marion JM: Neonatal progesterone and feminine sexual development. Nature 264:795–796, 1976.

Shearman RP, Garrett WJ: Double-blind study of effect of 17-hydroxyprogesterone caproate on abortion rate. Br Med J 1:292–295, 1963.

Snyder AM, Hull EM, Roth JA: The effect of maternal progesterone injections on fetal development of brain monoamine oxidase of rats. Brain Res 170:194–197, 1979.

Stehbens JA, Baker GL, Kitchell M: Outcome at ages 1, 3, and 5 years of children born to diabetic women. Am J Obstet Gynecol 127:408–413, 1977.

Tulchinsky D, Okada DM: Hormones in human pregnancy. IV. Plasma progesterone. Am J Obstet Gynecol 121:293–299, 1975.

Vande Wiele RL, Husami N, Dyrenfurth I: Progestogens in pregnancy. In New MI, Fiser RH Jr (eds): "Diabetes and other Endocrine Disorders During Pregnancy and in the Newborn." New York: Alan R Liss, Inc, 1976, pp 179–203.

Waber DP: Sex differences in cognition: A function of maturation rate? Science 192:572–574, 1976.

Waber DP: Sex differences in mental abilities, hemispheric lateralization, and rate of physical growth at adolescence. Dev Psychol 13:29–38, 1977.

Wilkins L: Masculinization of female fetus due to use of orally given progestins. JAMA 172:1028–1032, 1960.

Yalom ID, Green R, Fisk N: Prenatal exposure to female hormones. Arch Gen Psychiatry 28:554–561, 1973.

Zussman JU, Zussman PP, Dalton K: Post-pubertal effects of prenatal administration of progesterone. Presented at the Meeting of the Society for Research in Child Development. Denver, 1975.

Zussman JU, Zussman PP, Dalton K: Effects of prenatal progesterone on adolescent cognitive and social development. Presented at 3rd Annual Meeting of the International Academy of Sex Research Bloomington, 1977.

Neurobehavioral Effects of Prenatal Origin: Drugs of Use and Abuse

Donald E. Hutchings

Recently, I reviewed the behavioral teratology literature [1], and rather than use these pages to reiterate the clinical and animal findings in the area, I will attempt instead to define the field more precisely and to outline, at least from my point of view, some of the problems facing us as a new discipline.

Behavioral teratology represents an integration of teratology with experimental psychology and is primarily concerned with the study of neurobehavioral changes that result from exposure of germ cells, embryos, fetuses, and immature postnatal individuals to a variety of environmental disturbances and events. Like its parent discipline, teratology, these include drugs, industrial chemicals, pesticides, food additives and preservatives, and environmental pollutants, as well as irradiation, stress, infectious agents, and endocrine and metabolic disturbances [2]. Its major objective is the description of the behavioral effects induced by these conditions and an understanding of the embryopathic mechanisms by which they are produced. I should emphasize, however, the current state of behavioral teratology as a fledgling discipline; its subject matter remains largely unexplored and uncharted, its methodology is uneven and occasionally wanting, and its accomplishments strike a tenuous balance between false starts and palpable inroads made by a few pioneering researchers. But despite its immaturity and tentative beginnings, there should be no doubt that it is emerging as a new scientific specialty.

In my view [1] behavioral teratology belongs within the general theoretical framework of its parent discipline, teratology, and the paradigm of teratogenic action formulated by Wilson [2] provides a useful model for elucidating neurobehavioral effects. This scheme describes how teratogens initiate a sequence of

Drug and Chemical Risks to the Fetus and Newborn: 109–114

pathogenic effects beginning at the cellular level. Here, by interfering with some fundamental aspect of cellular physiology, such as protein synthesis or enzyme activity, these agents produce, for example, cell death or a failure of cellular interactions. Wilson suggests that ". . . these initially different types of pathogenesis may converge into a relatively narrow channel of abnormal development, for example, one that would lead ultimately to insufficient cells or cell products to carry out morphogenesis or to carry on function at the site of the final defect" [2, p 25].

In other words, an agent may have a very specific toxic action at the cellular level. It might, for example, kill actively proliferating cells while sparing those in the resting phase or only those cells in a particular phase of the cell cycle. In either case, however, populations of cells are killed and are therefore not available to participate in the developmental process. The final defect in the pathogenic sequence can include death, malformation, growth retardation, and neurobehavioral impairment.

Wilson has used this paradigm specifically to describe embryopathic mechanisms of teratogenic agents – that is, agents, in the strict sense, that cause gross structural defects. It is likely, however, that this same sort of paradigm applies to mechanisms of developmentally toxic nonteratogenic agents – agents that may cause growth retardation, neurobehavioral deficits, and in high doses, death, but not gross structural defects. These agents (eg, heroin and methadone, certain tranquilizers, stimulants, and hypnotics) may not selectively kill embryonic cells but, instead, exert their effect by interfering with neurochemical mechanisms in the developing brain. Though their action is poorly understood, some may act on specific embryonic sites (eg, synapses) or may interfere with the elaboration of neural systems utilizing particular neurotransmitters (eg, catecholamines) to initiate a sequence of abnormal development.

As animal research continues in this area and clinicians detect more clinical syndromes, we are beginning to appreciate the broad and complex range of neurobehavioral effects that can result from prenatal exposure to environmental substances. Among prescription drugs and substances of abuse known to be teratogenic in man, hydantoin [3] and alcohol (see chapter by Smith, this volume) each produce a syndrome in infants that includes a pattern of structural and behavioral defects that comprise abnormalities of growth, dysmorphic craniofacial features, and mental retardation.

On the other hand, neither heroin nor methadone appears to produce gross structural malformations in humans. Both, however, produce behavioral effects that occur in two phases; a neonatal withdrawal syndrome at birth characterized by tremors, hyperreflexia, irritability, excessive high-pitched crying, and disturbed sleep, and later, long-term neurobehavioral impairments that appear to include hyperactivity and short attention span.

Identification of these impairments and their suspected cause was aided by the severity of the symptoms seen during the neonatal period. In the case of alcohol and hydantoin, mental retardation occurs along with a unique syndrome of structural defects; and with opiates, the withdrawal syndrome can be so severe that it eventually led several clinicians to do follow-up studies to determine the possibility of long-term sequelae. What this implies, of course, is that if a behavioral impairment occurs without a concomitant structural defect, or does not become obvious until the child reaches school age, it is unlikely that a pediatrician or child psychiatrist would suspect a prenatal cause. Even worse, the questions that might suggest such an association would probably never be asked. Possibly, behavioral teratology has already had its thalidomide episode, but the effects remain undiscovered in the population.

The current dilemma is a paucity of prospective clinical data linking prenatal exposure to later behavioral effects and the difficulty of establishing such a relationship even with large-scale epidemiological studies. As Barnes [4] points out, attempts to establish a causal relationship between exogenous agents and gross structural defects present at birth poses formidable problems and, with respect to behavioral impairments, I would maintain that we face even greater problems.

First, Barnes points out that structural defects can be either genetically determined or result from a wide variety of environmental agents. And whether genetic or environmental, the defects, in most instances, are morphologically identical. Second, a particular environmental agent can produce a variety of defects that arise singly or as a syndrome, and with this lack of specificity it is difficult to establish in humans an unambiguous causal relationship. Barnes reminds us that the teratogenicity of thalidomide was discovered only because it produced such a rare syndrome of defects; more recently, alcohol was identified as a teratogen for the same reason. This lead Barnes to suggest that if thalidomide – or even aspirin – produced a more common type of defect like cleft palate or lip in, say, 5% of the cases in which it was consumed in the first trimester, it would probably not have been suspected. Or to put it the other way around, we are probably producing defective children all the time as a result of exposure to drugs and other compounds during the prenatal period. By the age of 1 year, 5–6% of children are recognized as having some sort of birth defect, which means that in a single year, as many as 250,000 defective children will be born in the United States. Barnes concludes that if prenatal exposure to teratogenic agents were responsible for 10,000–30,000 of these, and if they are the type of malformations that are also produced genetically, we would not even notice them.

Now apply this problem to attempts to establish a relationship between prenatal drug exposure and later neurobehavioral impairments. First, there is strong evidence indicating that at least some impairments, like gross structural defects, are of genetic origin but can also be produced by early exposure to environmental agents and, whether genetic or environmental, the symptomatology is virtually identical. For example, familial and genetic factors have been implicated as playing a significant role in the hyperkinetic syndrome [5], but this same behavioral impairment has also been reported in children following prenatal exposure to heroin, methadone [6–8], alcohol [9], and cigarette smoking [10]. A major problem is that hyperkinesis as well as other neurobehavioral symptoms such as short attention span, perceptual-motor impairments, coordination deficits, specific learning disabilities, and the like, are so prevalent and nonspecific as to obscure etiological identification. They are, if you will, the cleft lip and cleft palate of behavior.

Possibly, in order to implicate certain agents as causal, it will first be necessary to identify either unusual or extreme effects of syndromes both in animals and in man that are associated with a particular compound or drug (eg, barbiturates, amphetamines) or classes of drugs (eg, CNS depressants, stimulants). Then in order to establish an etiological relationship, there must follow a careful parallel comparison of both animal and human observations that generate testable hypotheses in both systems.

For example, the clinical reports that fetal exposure to methadone is associated with neurobehavioral deficits that persist into infancy and young childhood are difficult to interpret due to a host of confounding variables inherent in the population studied. The mothers frequently fail to obtain prenatal care, have poor diets, are heavy smokers, and many are concurrently using amphetamines, barbiturates, tranquilizers, or alcohol in a pattern of polydrug abuse. Moreover, the addicted neonate, depending upon the nature and severity of his withdrawal symptoms, is typically treated with paregoric, diazepam, chlorpromazine, or phenobarbitol. Adding to the confusion, the vast majority of the affected children come from the lower socioeconomic groups that are at risk, even when not exposed to drugs, for the same kinds of behavioral impairments seen among those exposed to methadone. Clearly, from clinical studies alone it is difficult to attribute, with any degree of confidence, these later deficits solely to prenatal methadone exposure.

Animal studies, however, have found behavioral effects very similar to those reported for humans. Exposing rats prenatally to morphine produces marked hyperactivity during the third and fourth postnatal weeks, followed by a return to the control level by 30 days of age [11]. We made similar observations in the young rat following prenatal methadone exposure and, in addition, found the hyperactivity to be associated with a disturbed sleep pattern [12]. Furthermore, during adulthood, though we found no evidence of a learning or inhibitory impairment on several operant-conditioning measures among methadone exposed offspring, they did develop extraordinarily high rates of response during particular phases of testing [13]. This suggested to us that the methadone-treated animals had a long-term neurobehavioral impairment characterized by the inability to modulate task-oriented motor output.

The possibility that hyperactivity and sleep disturbance would be observed in young animals following prenatal opiate exposure was suggested by clinical reports of human infants and children, and verifying the effect in young rats implicates opiates as causal in humans. Furthermore, the poorly modulated behavior found in the adult animal alerts the clinical practitioner and researcher alike to a particular kind of behavior problem that may emerge in the children as they reach maturity. This mutual trade-off cross-validates both the human and animal findings in a way that is impossible when the same observations are made independently and in isolation. The result is a powerful and meaningful set of comparative observations that relate prenatal drug effects to a general set of embryopathic and behavioral principles.

Prior to the recent research in behavioral teratology, studies of drug safety focused almost exclusively on early pregnancy – the time when the embryo is most vulnerable to serious structural damage. The health significance of malformations is, of course, obvious. They may be lethal, as in exencephaly, involve severe sensory disability such as deafness and blindness, or physical handicaps when limbs and digits fail to develop normally. The significance of behavioral teratologic studies is that they are providing compelling evidence demonstrating that developmentally toxic agents, by damaging or otherwise impairing CNS function, can have health consequences of equal import. These effects may be associated with hyperkinesis, attentional impairment, impulsivity, motor dysfunction, distractability, sleep disorders, learning disabilities, and, most serious, mental retardation.

Current research in this area is attempting to establish an effective methodology for studying the behavioral dimension of prenatal drug safety and provide some estimate of the potential hazard in the human population. It is hoped that these findings will alert the clinical practitioner to the kinds of neurobehavioral impairments that might be occurring in the human population and, if verified, lead to an effective program of prevention.

REFERENCES

1. Hutchings DE: Behavioral teratology: Embryopathic and behavioral effects of drugs during pregnancy. In Gottlieb G(ed): "Studies on the Development of Behavior and the Nervous System. Early Influences," Vol. 4. New York: Academic Press, 1978, pp 7–34.
2. Wilson JG: "Environment and Birth Defects." New York: Academic Press, 1973.
3. Hanson JW, Smith DW: Fetal hydantoin syndrome. Lancet 1:692, 1976.
4. Barnes AC: The fetal environment: Drugs and chemicals. In Barnes AC: (ed): "Intra-Uterine Development." Philadelphia: Lea & Febiger, 1968, pp 362–377.
5. Cantwell DP: Familial-genetic research with hyperactive children. In Cantwell DP (ed): "The Hyperactive Child." Holliswood, New York: Spectrum 1975, p 93.
6. Davis MM, Brown B, Glendinning S: Neonatal effects of heroin addiction and methadone-treated pregnancies. Preliminary report on 70 live births. In "Proceedings of the Fifth National Conference on Methadone Treatment." New York: National Association for the Prevention of Addiction to Narcotics, 1973, pp 1153–1164.
7. Ting R, Keller A, Berman P, Finnegan L: Follow-up studies of infants born to methadone-dependent mothers. Pediatr Res 8:346, 1974 (abstr).
8. Wilson G, Demond M, Verniaud W: Early development of infants of heroin-addicted mothers. Am J Dis Child 126:457, 1973.
9. Streissguth AP, Herman CS, Smith D: Intelligence, behavior and dymorphogenesis in the fetal alcohol syndrome: A report on 20 patients. J Pediatr 92:3, 1978.

10. Denson R, Nanson MA, McWatters MA: Hyperkinesis and maternal smoking. Can Psychiatr Assoc J 20: pp 183–187, 1975.
11. Sobrian SK: Prenatal morphine alters behavioral development in the rat. Pharmacol Biochem Behav 7:185, 1977.
12. Hutchings DE, Feraru E, Gorinson HS, Golden RR: Effects of prenatal methadone on the rest-activity cycle of the pre-weanling rat. Neurobehav Toxicol 1:33, 1979.
13. Hutchings DE, Towey JP, Gorinson HS, Hunt HF: Methodone during pregnancy: Assessment of behavior effects in the rat offspring. J Pharm Exp Ther 208:106, 1979.

The Excretion of Drugs in Human Milk

Cheston M. Berlin, Jr., MD

The breast combines the functions of the liver and kidney; it synthesizes and excretes. For a 4 kg infant requiring 100 kcal/kg/day, the mother easily makes 600 cc of milk containing 72 gm of protein, 22.2 gm of fat, 42 gm of carbohydrate (lactose), and appropriate concentration of minerals and vitamins. This product is delivered, on demand, sterile, and with the carbohydrate and protein suspended in a mineral/aqueous system. The fat is excreted as a milk fat globule, a spherical structure with a limiting lipoprotein membrane enclosing the lipid core. All nutrient components are fully digestible. Most research on lactation has been done in animals. There are quantitative differences between human and animal milk such as type of protein and pH (human 7.0 or above, cow 6.8 or below), but there is no reason to assume there are substantial qualitative differences in either milk formation or drug excretion.

The structure of the breast alveolar cell, which accomplishes all of this, is shown in Figure 1. Lactose is entirely synthesized from blood glucose in the breast alveolar cell. Its synthesis proceeds from UDP-galactose and glucose with lactose synthetase (galactose-transferase plus lactalbumin) as the enzyme. Prolactin is absolutely required. Lactose is excreted from the cell into the alveolar lumen alone with milk protein.

For fats, acetate is used for short chain fatty acids. Long chain fatty acids are supplied by transfer from plasma. Both classes of fat are esterified in the breast with glycerol (from intracellular glucose). The lipids collect in the endoplasmic reticulum. These lipids coalesce into droplets, which increase in size as they ascend the cell toward the lumen. As they ascend, they acquire a three-layered membrane (lipoprotein) and are extruded into milk (by reverse pinocytosis) as milk fat globules [1].

Drug and Chemical Risks to the Fetus and Newborn: 115–127

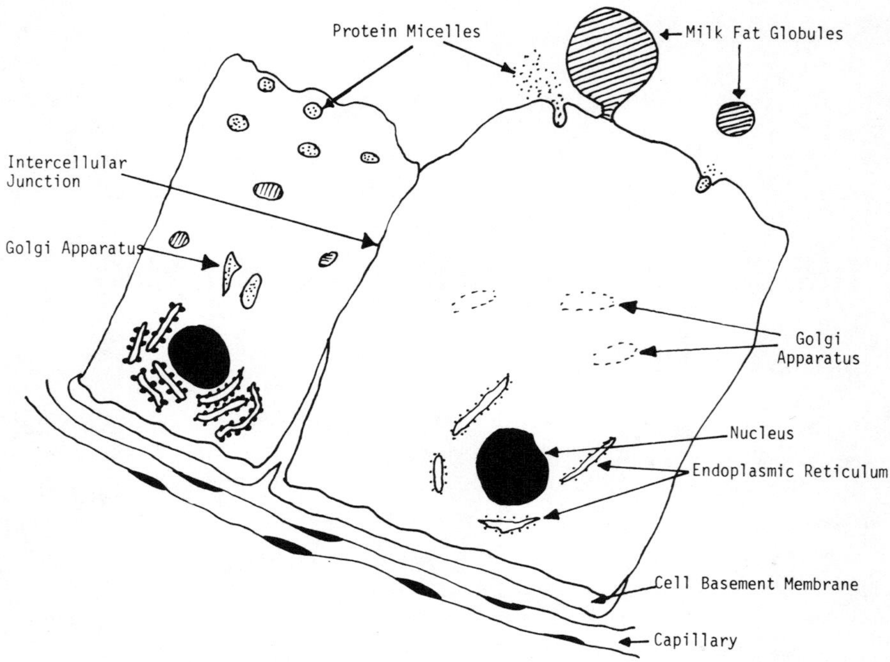

Fig. 1. Schematic drawing of alveolar breast cells. The cell on the left is actively synthesizing protein, fat and carbohydrate. The cell on the right has discharged most of the products into the alveolar lumen as milk. Carbohydrate is secreted with protein.

The milk proteins are fully synthesized within the cell from substrates delivered from the maternal circulation. Since these substrates cross the alveolar cell, it is reasonable to expect that other chemicals in maternal plasma, such as drugs, can also appear in breast milk. The major proteins are casein and lactalbumin (latter also needed for lactose synthesis). These proteins are very digestible and contribute to the low curd tension of human milk. The proteins are transported from the endoplasmic reticulum into the Golgi apparatus, migrate from the base of the cell toward the apex, and are discharged into the alveolar lumen via apocrine secretion.

Drug excretion into milk may be accomplished by binding to milk protein or to the surface of the milk fat globule. It is also possible that lipid-soluble drugs (eg DDT, PCB, insecticides) may be trapped entirely within the milk fat globule.

Rasmussen [2–4] has extensively studied drug excretion in animals (chiefly the cow and goat). His work is responsible for most of the current theories of drug excretion into milk. The most important factors seem to be 1) degree of ionization, 2) lipid solubility, and 3) molecular weight. As Figure 1 depicts, a drug must cross a number of structures before it appears in milk – capillary wall, interstitial water, breast alveolar cell wall, alveolar plasma membrane – and pass into, or bind to, any of intracellular structures prior to excretion into milk.

The drug may leave the cell by diffusion, reverse pinocytosis, or apocrine secretion (apical part of cell disintegrates). The entire process has been detailed by Vorherr [5].

In order for the drug to enter milk it must either traverse the breast alveolar cell or diffuse *between* alveolar cells (unlikely because of tight space between cells). Once the drug leaves the capillary, it may enter the alveolar cell by transcellular diffusion, passive diffusion in water filled channels, or by being bound to carrier proteins (ionophore diffusion).

Unionized molecules of small molecular weight appear to transverse the easiest into milk. Ethanol [6], urea [2], and antipyrine [7] have nearly identical simultaneous plasma and milk values.

The movement across a cell membrane of a partially ionized molecule obeys the Henderson-Hasselbach equation; this relationship has been extended to drug movement across the breast alveolar cell into milk. Knowing the degree of ionization of the drug (pK_a) plus the pH difference across the membrane, the milk/plasma (M/P) ratio can be calculated. This distribution has been well presented by Rasmussen [2]. Figure 2 illustrates the distribution of two weakly acid drugs with

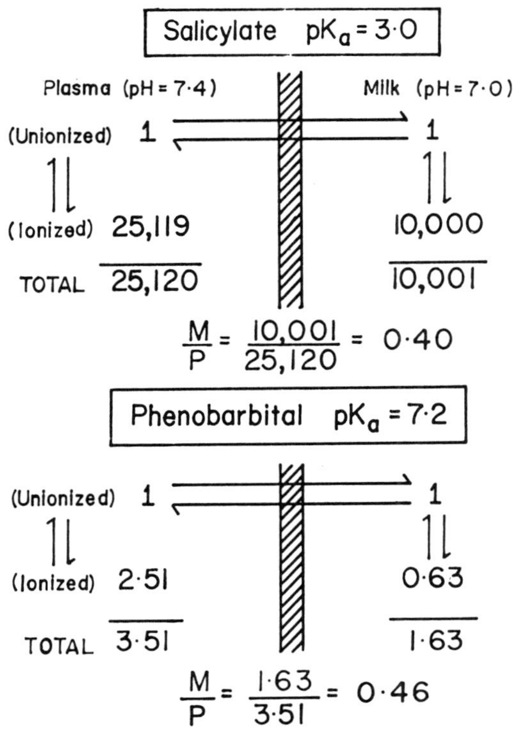

Fig. 2. Theoretical distribution across a semipermeable membrane of two weakly acidic drugs with different pK_as: salicylate (pK_a = 3.0) and phenobarbital (pK_a = 7.2).

markedly different pK_as: salicylic acid ($pK_a = 3.0$) and phenobarbital ($pK_a = 7.2$). Plasma pH is assumed to be 7.4, and milk pH, 7.0. For a weak acid at equilibrium, the ratio of un-ionized (U) to ionized (I) drug is:

$$\log \frac{U}{I} = pK_a - pH$$

For a weak base
$$\log \frac{I}{U} = pK_a - pH$$

Theoretical M/P ratio for total salicylate (un-ionized plus ionized) is 0.40; the experimental value obtained by Miller et al [8] is 0.35. The theoretical ratio for total phenobarbital is 0.46; the experimental value is 0.7 [3]. The difference for phenobarbital may be explained by the significant lipid solubility of this drug (chloroform/water distribution of un-ionized drug = 4.8). Thus the presence on one side of a biological membrane of a substance rich in fat (milk) will introduce another factor in the final determination of the concentration of a drug in breast milk.

Drugs with little ionization and a high degree of lipid solubility cross cell membranes easily [9]. This is of great current concern because of certain environmental chemicals that appear to be taken up by body fat. Lactation may be the only route of elimination for these compounds [10]. Such chemicals include tetrahydrocannibinol (no human data), polyhalogenated biphenyls (PBB and PCB) [10], DDT [11], and other insecticides. The safe limit of these agents is simply not known. Mothers in Michigan with detectable levels of PBBs in their milk nursed infants with no apparent deleterious effect. Women in the childbearing age should avoid exposure to these compounds. If any question arises, measurement of the chemical should be made in milk samples from the nursing mother.

Compounds with a molecular weight greater than 200 do not cross membranes well [2]. There exist many tables [12–17] of the concentration of a drug in human milk following maternal ingestion. In few drugs has distribution and excretion been studied in a systematic fashion. The concentrations given in these tables are measured at only one time point after maternal administration and that time varies considerably, not only from drug to drug, but also in different studies of the same drug.

For this reason antipyrine distribution was studied in nursing mothers who were weaning their infants, or were able to postpone nursing for eight or more hours (to minimize infant exposure to antipyrine) [7]. At 0900, six lactating women were given 18 mg/kg antipyrine orally. Simultaneous milk and saliva samples were ob-

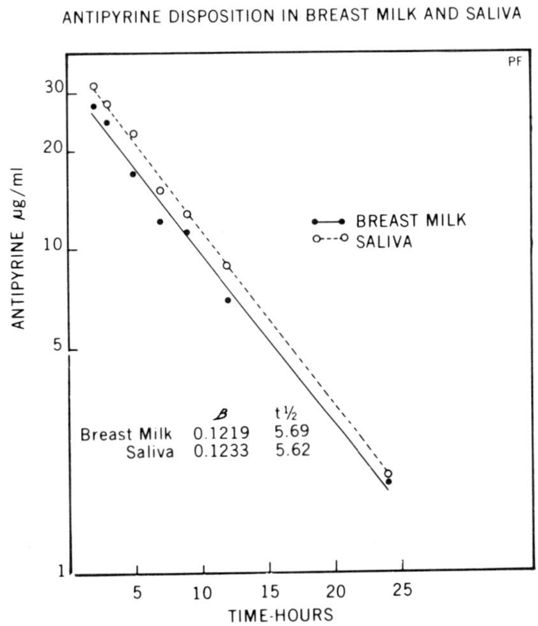

Fig. 3. Concentration of antipyrine in the saliva and milk of a lactating woman. Antipyrine (18 mg/kg) was given in a single oral dose at 0 hours.

tained at 0, 1, 2, 3, 5, 7, 9, 12, 24, and 48 hours. The saliva/plasma ratio for antipyrine is 1, thus obviating the need for venipunctures. Figure 3 shows the data from one patient. There was prompt appearance of antipyrine in milk (by ten minutes in two patients in which multiple samples were obtained in the first hour after antipyrine). Levels of antipyrine in milk were very similar to the simultaneously measured saliva (and hence plasma) levels. The milk/saliva ratio for the data points in Figure 3 varied from 0.76 to 0.90. The elimination rate constants for both milk (0.1219 hr^{-1}) and saliva (0.1233 hr^{-1}) were very similar and hence were the half-lives (5.69 hours in milk and 5.62 hours in saliva). Data from the other five mothers showed similar close correspondence between saliva (plasma) and milk appearance and elimination.

How much antipyrine would be available to the infant through mother's milk? Assume the infant will nurse 200 cc every four hours for the 24 hours after antipyrine. This is a generous figure and would certainly represent the upper limit. Table I shows the data for all six mothers. The total amount available ranged from 6.6 to 24.7 mg or 0.56% to 2.38% of maternal dose. This is one figure that is needed for all drugs to properly assess risk to the nursing infant.

TABLE I. Amount of Antipyrine Available to a Nursing Infant Assuming the Infant Nurses 200 cc Every Four Hours After Maternal Antipyrine Administration (18mg/kg in a single oral dose)

Mother	Antipyrine (mg)	% Maternal dose
1	6.6	0.56
2	9.8	0.96
3	12.0	0.87
4	12.8	1.30
5	21.1	1.97
6	24.7	2.38

Sulfasalazine (Azulfidine) is a drug recently studied [18] in our laboratory that illustrates some of the points regarding drug excretion into milk. The opportunity for study arose because a nursing mother needed to take this drug for control of ulcerative colitis. Sulfasalazine is a drug composed of the sulfonamide sulfapyridine, coupled to a salicylate, 5-aminosalicylic acid. Its molecular weight is 398.4. Sulfasalazine is cleaved by gut bacteria to its two constituents 5-aminosalicylate and sulfapyridine. The latter drug undergoes N-acetylation and 5 hydroxylation followed by conjugation of both compounds with glucuronic acid. The patient received 500 mg of sulfasalazine every six hours orally. A total of 44 milk samples collected over a 3-month period were studied, with occasional urine, saliva and plasma samples. Although the parent drug, sulfasalazine, readily appeared in the mother's plasma and urine (her plasma and urine were grossly orange), it was undetectable in all milk samples. Its high molecular weight no doubt limited its transport into milk. 5-Aminosalicylate is usually not detected in the human plasma, the very low levels being rapidly cleared by the kidney. Hence this drug was not detected in mother's plasma, saliva, or milk. Sulfapyridine and its metabolites were all detected in both plasma and milk at fairly constant levels (4–7 μg/ml). Assuming a continual milk level for 5 μg/ml, the 24-hour dose available to the infant was 4 mg, or about 0.32% of the maternal oral dose of sulfapyridine in the form of sulfasalazine. Random urine samples from the infant showed a 24-hour urinary excretion of about 2 mg, or 50% of the delivered dose. This amount (2 mg/day) does not appear to be hazardous to the nursing infant in absence of sulfonamide allergy.

These two drugs illustrate the kind of information needed to assess the risk to the nursing infant. Table II is a list of drugs for which data exist in the literature to calculate, as the last column indicates, the total amount excreted by the mother. It is usually less than 1–2% of the maternal dose. Clearly, many other drugs need to be thoroughly studied to assess their safety during lactation.

There is one area of critical importance for which virtually no data exist. Can the breast, which can so easily synthesize one liter per day of milk with all necessary constituents, metabolize drugs? It is most important to know if potentially toxic metabolites can be made in breast tissue and released into milk. In the antipyrine study described previously no metabolites of antipyrine were identified. In the sulfasalazine study, only those metabolites of sulfapyridine in maternal serum were identified in milk. However, it is important to continue searching for potentially toxic metabolites, especially in mothers on chronic drug therapy.

The list of drugs that a nursing mother ought not take (or if she must take them she ought not nurse) is given in Table III. Lithium easily crosses into milk; the nursling's plasma level may be one-third to one-half that of the mother. The anti-cancer drugs, as well as isoniazid, interfere with nucleic acid function. Isoniazid, besides its anti-DNA properties, can cause liver damage. This liver damage is apparently dependent on the formation of acetylisoniazid. This latter compound is excreted in breast milk [23]. Phenindione has been documented to cause bleeding, with prolonged prothrombin and partial thromboplastin times [41]. Chloramphenicol and propylthiouracil, both of which are found in milk after maternal ingestion, are included in this list because of their potential for depressing bone marrow function. Nursing should be avoided following administration of radioactive pharmaceuticals (usually used for diagnostic purposes). Table IV quantitates the potential exposure of the infant following maternal administration of three commonly used isotopes. Nursing may be resumed after 48 hours following technectium 99; a wait of two to three weeks is advisable after iodine 131 or gallium 67. Milk should be counted for radioactivity before nursing is resumed.

Note that the list of proscribed drugs (Table III) is quite small considering the vast array of therapeutic agents available. *This does not mean all others are safe; it usually means that insufficient evidence is available.* The analysis of drugs as listed in Table II indicates that the total drug available to nursing infants will be quite small (less than 1–2% of maternal dose). Assuming absence of toxic metabolites and drug allergy, the effect on the infant will probably not be evident by any means we currently have available.

For the nursing mother *no* drug administration is obviously best. For the occasional use of some drugs (*not* those in Table III), the amount available to the nursing infant can be minimized by taking the drug just after a feed and allowing as long as possible (four hours preferably) until the next feed. For mothers needing chronic therapy, much more knowledge is needed. The analysis of milk, as illustrated in the two examples given, can be used whenever a question of safety arises over drug therapy in a lactating mother. We must make breast feeding as safe as possible.

TABLE II. Drugs Excreted in Breast Milk

Drug [reference]	Maternal dose	μg/ml Peak level	M/P[a] ratio at peak
Antipyrine [7]	18 mg/kg	20–30	1.0
Cefazolin [19]	2 gm IV 500 mg IM tid	1.51 0	0.023
Chlorothiazide [20]	500 mg po Single dose		
Diazepam [21]	Not stated	0.27	0.68
Digoxin [22]	0.25 mg	0.6–1.0 ng/ml	0.8–0.9
Ethanol [6]	0.6 gm/kg	777	0.93
Isoniazid [23]	300 mg	16.6	1.6
Lithium [24]	Chronic; dose not specified	0.1–0.6 mmole/liter	0.5
Methadone [25]	70 mg/day	0.36 0.51	0.83 1.89
Nicotine [26]	1 pack/day 400 mg	91 ng/ml range 20–512	
Prednisolone [27]	5 mg	26 ng/ml	
Prednisone [28]	120 mg	154 ng/ml (prednisone) 473 ng/ml (prednisolone)	
Propranolol [29]	20 mg 160 mg	10 ng/ml 150 ng/ml	0.56 0.65
Salicylate [30]	20 mg/kg		
Sulfasalazine [18]	2 gm/day (chronic)	9–15 mg/ml (as sulfapyridine)	0.8
Sulphone [31]		14	0.16
Theophylline [32]	4.25 mg/kg	4 μg/ml	0.7

[a]M/P = milk/plasma ratio.

[b]$t_{1/2}$ is calculated from the elimination (β) phase.

[c]Amount excreted in 24 hours is estimated by assuming the infant ingests 90 cc of milk every four hours.

[d]The % of maternal dose is calculated by dividing the amount secreted in 24 hours by the maternal dose (single dose or 24-hour total maternal dose).

Time of peak level	$t_{1/2}$[b]	Amount secreted in 24° after single dose[c]	% Maternal dose[d]
10 minutes	6–22 hours	7–25 mg	0.5–2:4
3 hours		1.5 mg	0.075
Not detected in milk		0	
Not detected in milk (<1 μg/ml)		< 1 mg/day	
3 days	3 days	0.27 mg (peak) on day 3	
4 hours	12 hours	0.18–0.36 μg/day	0.07–0.14
90 minutes	2.9 hours	300 mg	1
3 hours	5.9 hours	7 mg	2.3
Levels fairly constant			
		300 μg	
No correlation		0.68 mg	0.17
1 hour	8.2 hours	6 μg	0.12
2 hours	1.8 hours	47 μg (as both prednisone and prednisolone)	0.04
2 hours	1.1 hours		
3 hours		0.6 μg	0.03
3 hours		90 μg	0.05
			0.18–0.36
Constant level		1.4–2.1 mg	0.16
6 hours		10 mg	2
2 hours	4.0 hours	8 mg	4

TABLE III. Drugs Contraindicated in the Nursing Mother

Drug [reference]	Reason
Lithium [24]	Significant blood levels in the infant (1/3–1/2 maternal levels)
INH [23]	Anti-DNA drug; metabolite (acetyl INH) which is thought responsible for liver toxicity in milk
Antimetabolites [33]	Anti-DNA activity
Radioactive pharmaceuticals [34–36]	Radioactivity present in breast milk (see Table IV)
Very lipid soluble drugs [37–40] (hexachlorophene, PBCs, DDT, THC)	Only elimination route through milk; measure level if any doubt of maternal body burden
Phenindione [41]	Bleeding in one case report with ↑PT and ↑PTT
Mothers homozygous for cystic fibrosis [42]	Sodium content of milk high: 132–280 mEq/liter
Chloramphenicol	Possible bone marrow depression
Propylthiouracil	Possible goiter and bone marrow suppression

TABLE IV. Secretion of Radioactive Isotopes in Milk*

Isotope [reference]	Maternal dose	$t_{1/2}$	Amount in milk (μCi/ml)	Infant dose (μCi/day)	Cumulative dose to infant (μCi)
^{67}Ga [58]	3 mCi IC	78 hours	3 days 0.15	75	350 (if nursed from day 3 on)
			7 days 0.045	23	108 (if nursed from day 7 on)
			14 days 0.010	5	23 (if nursed from day 14 on)
^{131}I [59]	200 μCi IV	24 hours	25 hours 0.028	6	15 (if nursed through day 5) 7.5% of maternal dose
^{99m}Tc [60]	15 mCi IV	4 hours	8.5 hours 0.1	95	0.63% of maternal dose
			20 hours 0.02		
			60 hours 0.006		

*The data in the last two columns are calculated by assuming the infant takes 3 ounces of breast milk every four hours.

REFERENCES

1. Patton S, Keenan TW: The milk fat globule membrane. Biochim Biophys Acta 415: 273, 1975.
2. Rasmussen F: Excretion of drugs by milk. In Brodie BB, Gilette JR (eds): "Handbook of Experimental Pharmacology," Vol. 28. "Concepts in Biochemical Pharmacology," Part I. New York: Springer-Verlag, 1971, p 390.
3. Rasmussen F: Students on the mammary excretion and absorption of drugs. Copenhagen: C. Fr. Martenson, 1966.
4. Rasmussen F: The mechanisms of drug secretion into milk. In Galli G, Jacini G, Pecile A (eds): "Dietary Lipids and Postnatal Development." New York: Raven Press, 1973, p 231.
5. Vorherr H: "The Breast." New York: Academic Press, 1974, p 107.
6. Kesaniema YA: Ethanol and acetaldehyde in the milk and peripheral blood of lactating women after ethanol administration. J Obst Gynecol Br Commonw 81:84, 1974.
7. Berlin CM: Antipyrine appearance and decay in human breast milk and saliva. Pharmacologist 20:219, 1978.
8. Miller GE, Banejee NC, Stowie CM Jr: Drug movement between bovine milk and plasmá as affected by milk pH. J Dairy Sci 50:1395, 1967.
9. Schanker LS: Passage of drugs across body membranes. Pharmacol Rev 14:501, 1962.
10. Brilliant LB, Amburg GV, Isbister J, Humphrey H, Wilcox K, Eyster J, Bloomer AW, Price H: Breast-milk monitoring to measure Michigan's contamination with polybrominated biphenyls. Lancet 2:643, 1978.
11. Kroger M: Insecticide residues in human milk. J Pediatr 80:401, 1972.
12. Knowles JA: Excretion of drugs in milk – A review. Pediatrics 66:1068, 1965.
13. Savage RL: Drugs and Breast Milk Adverse Drug Reaction Bulletin (Pub. by Regional Postgraduate Institute for Medicine and Dentistry, Newcastle upon Tyne). No. 61, 212, 1976.
14. Rivera-Calimlim L: Drugs in breast milk. Drug Therapy December:59, 1977.
15. Hervada AR, Feit E, Sagrames R: Drugs in breast milk. Perinat Care 2:19, 1978.
16. O'Brien TE: Excretion of drugs in human milk. Am J Hosp Pharm 31:844, 1974.
17. Catz CS, Giacoia GP: Drugs and breast milk. Pediatr Clin North Am 19:151, 1972.
18. Berlin CM, Yaffe SJ: Disposition of sulfasalazine (azulfidine) in human breast milk, plasma, and saliva. Pediatr Res 13:396, 1979.
19. Yoshioka H, Cho K, Takimoto M, Maruyama S, Shimzu T: Transfer of cefazolin into human milk. J Pediatr 94:151, 1979.
20. Werthmann MW, Krees SV: Excretion of chlorothiazide in human breast milk. J Pediatr 81:781, 1972.
21. Cole AP, Hailey DM: Diazepam and active metabolite in breast milk and their transfer to the neonate. Arch Dis Child 50:741, 1975.
22. Loughnan PM: Digoxin excretion in human breast milk. J Pediatr 92:1019, 1978.
23. Berlin CM, Lee C: Isoniazid and acetylisoniazid disposition in human milk, saliva and plasma. Fed Proc 38:426, 1979.
24. Schou M, Amdisen A: Lithium and pregnancy – III, Lithium ingestion by children breast fed by women on lithium treatment. Br Med J 2:138, 1973.
25. Blinick G, Inturrisi CE, Jerez E, Wallach RC: Methadone assays in pregnant women and progeny. Am J Obstet Gynecol 121:617, 1975.
26. Ferguson BB, Wilson DJ, Schaffner W: Determination of nicotine concentrations in human milk. Am J Dis Child 130:837, 1976.

27. McKenzie SA, Selley JA, Agnew JE: Secretion of prednisolone into breast milk. Arch Dis Child 50:894, 1975.
28. Berlin CM, Demers L, Kaiser D: Prednisone and prednisolone in human milk after large oral dose of prednisone. Pharmacologist. 21:26, 1979.
29. Karlberg B, Lindberg D, Aberg H: Excretion of propranolol in human breast milk. Acta Pharmacol Toxicol 34:222, 1974.
30. Levy G: Salicylate pharmacokinetics in the human neonate. In Morselli PL, Garactini G, Sereni F (eds): "Basic and Therapeutic Aspects of Perinatal Pharmacology." New York: Raven Press, 1975, p 319.
31. Dreisbach JA: Sulphone levels in breast milk of mothers on sulphone therapy. Lebrosy Review 23:101, 1952.
32. Yurchak AM, Jusko WJ: Theophylline secretion into breast milk. Pediatrics 57:518, 1976.
33. Wienick PH, Duncan JH: Cyclophosphamide in human milk. Lancet 1:912, 1971.
34. Tobin RE, Schneider PB: Uptake of ^{67}Ga in the lactating breast and its persistence in milk: Case report. J Nucl Med 17:1055, 1976.
35. Wyburn JR: Human breast milk excretion of radionuclides following administration of radiopharmaceuticals. J Nucl Med 14:115, 1973.
36. Rumble WF, Aamodt RL, Jones AE, Henkin RI, Johnston GS: Accidental ingestion of Tc-99m in breast milk by a 10-week-old child. J Nucl Med 19:913, 1978.
37. Laug EP, Kunze FM, Prickett CS: Occurrence of DDT in human fat and milk. Arch Ind Hyg Occup Med 3:245, 1951.
38. WHO/FAO. Pesticide Residues in Food. Technical Report Series No. 417, Geneva, 1969.
39. Brenik EM, Bjerk JE: Organochlorine compounds in Norwegian human fat and milk. Acta Pharmacol Toxicol 43:59, 1978.
40. Bakken, Arne F, Seip M: Insecticides in human breast milk. Acta Paediatr Scand 65: 535, 1976.
41. deSweet M, Lewis PJ: Excretion of anticoagulants in human milk. N Engl J Med 297: 1471, 1977.

The Contamination of the Food Chain in Michigan With PBB: The Breast-Feeding Question

Ronald L. Poland, MD, and Sanford N. Cohen, MD

Polybrominated biphenyls (PBBs) were accidentally introduced into the human food chain throughout the lower peninsula of the state of Michigan in mid-1973. By 1976, a survey of women in Michigan revealed widespread contamination of human milk samples with PBB. The survey alarmed state officials. The contaminated milk was seen as a potential health hazard to infants in the state. Guidelines were needed to provide women in Michigan with appropriate advice on the question of nursing their infants. This report details the events leading up to the Michigan Department of Public Health advisory on breast feeding [December, 1976] and the process used to develop the position taken. Many of the historical events recounted here come from newspaper coverage at the time. The remainder of this account results from personal involvement on the advisory committees, a review of the literature on PBB, and interviews with some investigators still working on the follow-up projects.

HISTORY

In late 1972 and early 1973 a paper shortage existed in the United States. Many people were hoarding paper products in their homes, and Johnny Carson was making the most of the humorous side of the inconvenience. At that time two products,

Drug and Chemical Risks to the Fetus and Newborn: 129–137

"Firemaster" and "Nutrimaster," were manufactured by the same Michigan-based chemical company. The company's usual procedure was to ship "Firemaster BP-6" only with the respective brand names. The former was a mixture of polybrominated biphenyls used as a flame retardant in the manufacture of thermoplastics, and the latter was magnesium oxide, a nutrient additive for cattle feed.

In May 1973, "Firemaster" was packaged and shipped in brown bags because red ones were temporarily unobtainable. It is alleged that some or all of a shipment of what was thought to have been magnesium oxide to a major Michigan feed mill was really the polybrominated biphenyl mixture (PBB).* The PBB was pelleted into a major batch of cattle feed in concentrations of up to 4,300 ppm and distributed. This fact remained undiscovered for another year.

In October 1973, some herds of cattle in Michigan were observed to develop an illness. They refused their feed, lost weight, and milk production decreased. Many became lame with an abnormal hoof growth. Both cattle and swine exhibited increased abortion rates, and heifers failed to breed. Enlarged livers were seen in 100 cattle coming to slaughter. Some farmers became concerned and asked the Michigan Department of Agriculture for advice. No useful advice could be given. One of the farmers suspected the feed and sent samples of feed to a laboratory for independent chemical analysis. PBB was identified in the feed.

In May 1974, the Michigan Department of Public Health (DPH) took action to stop the spread of PBB in the food chain of the state. State tolerances were established according to existent federal guidelines (derived from limited animal studies) and then were reduced further by the state as technology improved. In May 1974, the state banned the sale of milk or meat with fat concentrations of PBB above 1.0 ppm (μg/gm fat), and in November 1974 this tolerable level was reduced to 0.3 ppm. Over 500 farms were quarantined. Livestock (30,000) and poultry (1.6 million) were destroyed. Contaminated animal feed (788 tons), butter (3,000 lb), cheese (18,000 lb), dry milk (34,000 lb) and eggs (5 million) were buried [1].

In the summer and fall of 1974, DPH initiated studies to learn the extent of the human exposure to PBB. PBB blood levels of residents of quarantined farms ranged up to 2.26 ppm and those of residents of non-quarantined farms up to 0.02 ppm. Adipose tissue levels were found to average 170 times that of blood; breast milk fat levels were about 100 times that of paired blood samples. The state surveys showed that almost all breast milk samples obtained from inhabitants of quarantined farms exceeded the tolerance level set for bovine milk and that half of the samples obtained from other women in the state had more than 0.07 ppm PBB (Tables I and II). Since breast-fed infants may receive no other source of calories, some authorities considered that tolerance levels to be set for human milk might have to be lower than for bovine milk. The Michigan Department of Public Health, therefore, considered strongly the banning of breast feeding in the state.

*An employee of the feed mill claimed to have questioned the change in labeling on the bags and to have been told not to use them. His supervisor recalls no such conversation.

Table I. Survey of PBB Concentrations (μg/gm of milk fat) in Samples From Women Throughout the Lower Peninsula of Michigan*

If a woman has level of PBB in fat of breast milk (ppm),	then the approximate % of lower peninsula women	
	having levels less than hers is:	having levels greater than hers is:
0.05 ppm	30%	70%
0.07 ppm	50%	50%
0.10 ppm	65%	35%
0.30 ppm	87%	13%
0.50 ppm	94%	6%
1.00 ppm	98%	2%

*Data from MDPH survey

TABLE II. PBB Levels in Milk Samples From Mothers From Quarantined Farms

		PBB levels (ppm)	
Subject	Date	Breast milk	Blood plasma
E.B.	12/74	10.800	0.082
C.M.	6/74	22.700	0.252
D.S.	10/74	1.800	0.014
L.H.	3/75	.210	0.003
S.S.	3/75	92.660	1.068

A proposed health advisory notice was composed, printed, and stuffed into envelopes for distribution to all of the physicians in the state. Before the scheduled mailing, a small committee of physicians and toxicologists was gathered outside the state capital to advise the director of the health department about the impact of such a ban. This ad hoc committee was composed primarily of pediatricians and obstetricians from schools of medicine and osteopathy in the state. The committee argued that:

1) The analogy used between mother's milk and commerical formulae was not altogether pertinent to the problem at hand.

2) The unique benefits of breast feeding were not being considered in the decision.

3) Comparably "toxic" levels of PCBs identified in milk samples all over the country had not prompted similar action anywhere.

4) The DPH would never have taken such an action against a large, legally protected, milk-producing company without better information, and

5) The information based upon laboratory animal data which was available and upon which they were acting was insufficient to justify so drastic a step.

Distribution of the health advisory was consequently postponed, and a panel of experts was assembled to weigh the risks and benefits of breast feeding in Michigan in light of the PBB contamination.

The select panel met on October 14, 1976, to review the breast milk survey and make recommendations for nursing mothers in Michigan. Included were pediatricians and obstetricians from Michigan, representatives of the American Academy of Pediatrics, the Food and Drug Administration, the National Cancer Foundation, the Center for Disease Control, and the LaLeche League.*

ANALYSIS OF DATA AVAILABLE BY OCTOBER 1976

An article by Kay summarizes much of the relevant information about PBB available by October 1976 [2]. PBB was known to cause severe systemic illness in cattle fed large doses in contaminated diets (4,000–13,500 ppm for 6–18 months [3]. A diet that contained 50 ppm produced no ill effects in cattle when fed for 60 days [4]. Chickens fed PBB in their regular diet (5, 10, and 20 ppm) for 8 weeks showed no ill effects, but a diet containing 45 ppm did cause diminished egg production [5,6].

Almost all of the rodent species tested showed induction of hepatic enzymes analogous to that caused by phenobarbitol and a number of other environmental contaminants even when only 1.0 ppm was added to the feed [7]. Some studies have suggested that PBB (50 and 100 ppm) may be teratogenic in rodents, but others have not [2]. Corbet and his co-workers [8], concluded that PBB was "weakly teratogenic" in rodents. A careful review of that paper indicated that the "statistically significant" data included a large number of control animals from another laboratory. When the concomitant control animals from the investigator's laboratory were compared with the PBB-fed animals, there was no apparent difference in the outcome between the two groups.

There are wide differences between various animal species in their threshold to specific toxic effects of PBB. Up to the fall of 1976, no deleterious effect had been noted in any species when the diet contained less than 2.0 ppm of PBB. Hepatic enzyme induction was the only change reported by an investigator who fed PBB in lower concentrations. There was no evidence of carcinogenesis or mutagenesis due to PBB. The data on teratogenesis were meager and showed no conclusive adverse effect.

More than 250 persons who were exposed to very high levels of PBB on quarantined farms were interviewed, examined, and studied for more than two and a half years. No simple relationship was found between even extreme PBB exposure and disease in man, although many people in the state were convinced that families on contaminated farms did suffer adverse effects on their health (such as alopecia,

*The panel members were Mel Barclay, MD, Audrey K. Brown, MD, Frank Cordle, PhD, Laurence Finberg, MD, Gary Flamm, MD, Renate D. Kimbrough, MD, Herman Kraybill, MD, Walter Meester, MD, PhD, Ronald L. Poland, MD, Herbert Ratner, MD and William B. Weil, Jr., MD.

lethargy, weakness, joint pains) caused by PBB [9]. Follow-up studies were continuing to look for possible long-term human toxicity of PBB.

ANALYSIS OF BREAST FEEDING PROBLEMS

Prevention

The select committee concluded that since all evidence suggested that PBB crosses the placenta freely, there was no way to prevent the exposure of infants born to women who had a body burden of PBB. Furthermore, the PBB levels in the fat of the fetus were likely to be similar to those in maternal fat. Breast-feeding under such circumstances would not initiate the exposure to the chemical, but it would prolong the exposure.

Estimate of Body Burden of PBB in Nursing Infants

The panel decided to construct a "worst case" model to evaluate the extra body burden of PBB accrued by nursing infants. The concentration of PBB in body fat (where the chemical is concentrated) of a newborn infant whose mother was at the sixty-fifth percentile for PBB concentration in milk (September–October 1976) was estimated to be 0.30 (Table III) ppm. The half-life of PBB in human fat after prolonged high dose exposure was estimated at about seven months, according to some preliminary data [Meester 1976, personal communication]. The half-life of PBB in cattle was reported to be 10½ days following low-dose exposure for 15 days [10] and almost two months following 50 ppm for 60 days [11]. Thus, finite disappearance rates were known for this material from the fat of individuals contaminated with it, and the concentration in milk was likely to fall in proportion to the fall in its concentration in other body fat stores.

Table III. Hypothetical Case

Assumptions:

1. Birthweight: 3.5 kg
   Fat content: 13%
   PBB content: 0.3 ppm (fat basis)
2. Breast feeding only × 5 months
   Milk PBB: 0.1 ppm (65th%)
   Fat intake: 5,042 gm
3. Weight at 5 months: 7 kg
   Fat content: 25%

Age	Body weight (kg)	Body fat (gm)	PBB content (μg)	PBB concentration (ppm)
Birth	3.5	450	135	0.30
5 months	7.0	1750	636	0.35
12 months	10.0	2134	636	0.30

Even if one assumed that 1) there was no excretion of PBB from either nursing mother or infant, 2) a constant 0.1 ppm would be excreted in the milk throughout a five-month period, and 3) all of the calories consumed by the infant during the five-month period would be provided by the contaminated breast milk; the concentration in the infant's fat might be predicted to increase from an original 0.30 ppm over the five months involved (Table II). Thus, even when unreasonably maximized assumptions are made, it was obvious that the concentration of PBB in the tissues of a nursing infant would not increase substantially due to breast feeding. In fact, the concentration of PBB might decrease early during the nursing period, even though the total body burden of the compound increased slightly.

Risk versus Benefit

The risk of feeding low level PBB contaminated material to young infants was not known but, on the basis of available information, the panel assumed it to be very small. The panel felt it wise to avoid feeding such material to an infant if there were alternative feeding mixtures that had the same nutritive and other qualities as breast milk. Breast milk, however, was known to have unique nutritional and immunological properties that are unmatched by any other milk or commercial product. Furthermore, the psychological advantages of breast feeding to both mother and infant were established well enough to add substantially to the benefit side of the equation.

The panel concluded that the benefits that accrue to an infant from breast feeding far outweigh the best estimate of the potential risk of continuing PBB exposure beyond the date of birth.

Additional Consideration

A number of chemical contaminants had been found in human milk samples in and out of the state several years before the PBB episode in Michigan. These chemicals included PCP, DDT, and others less widely known. No evidence had accumulated to connect any of these environmental contaminants of human milk to the production of human disease of any sort in nursing infants. Moreover, no suggestion was made by any authority in this field that women with such contaminants in their milk discontinue breast feeding their babies. The potential risks of feeding infants with PBB-contaminated human milk were evaluated more extensively than had the potential risks of feeding many of the other known contaminants. Thus, breast feeding was not discouraged among women in Michigan, in spite of the widespread distribution of PBB in human milk. Certain women who were suspected of having very high concentrations of PBB in their milk, either through extensive exposure to the chemical or by actual chemical determination, were encouraged to seek alternate feeding regimes for their infants.

The DPH responded to the recommendations of the select panel by canceling the distribution of the original health advisory letter. Instead, another letter was sent to the physicians of Michigan on December 20, 1976, which advised them of the findings of the select panel and announced that lactating women could have their milk analyzed for PBB level, if they wished, at state expense. The DPH has continued to support further research into the effects of PBB on humans and laboratory animals.

AFTERMATH

Since December 1976 more than 100 articles have been published on the effects of PBB on humans, laboratory animals, and the environment. Volume 23 of "Environmental Health Perspectives" (April 1978) was devoted entirely to PBB. Much of the data collected from residents of Michigan remains to be analyzed and interpreted. The volume of literature on the subject is likely to increase substantially in the next year or two. The following are some relevant studies that have been reported since the DPH breast-feeding advisory. We selected them for presentation because they have a tendency to contradict some of the assumptions made by the 1976 panel or because they present human outcomes not then available.

In 1978 Allen and co-workers [12] reported that a diet containing 0.3 ppm of PBB fed over a 7-month period to adult female rhesus monkeys was associated with a 7% weight loss and a lengthening of the menstrual cycle (in 4 of 7 animals). When the seven rhesus females were bred (after 66 weeks on the diet), five offspring resulted. A comparison of the birthweight and subsequent growth of the nursing monkeys with seven controls (not exposed to PBB before or after birth), showed that the PBB-exposed animals were smaller at birth and grew less rapidly up to 16 weeks of age (Fig. 1). PBB concentrations were not measured in blood, tissue, or milk in their study.

Immunologic studies have been carried out on farm residents in Michigan and Wisconsin by Bekesi and co-workers [13]. Forty percent of the 45 Michigan farm residents tested had lymphocyte populations with significantly reduced reactivity to phytohemaglutinin and pokeweed mitogen. Lymphocytes collected from all of the Michigan-based subjects exhibited significantly less (26–74% of control values) reactivity in mixed lymphocyte cultures. These investigators also noted fewer T-cells and B-cells, along with an increase in the number and percentage of null-cells, among the lymphocytes in the peripheral blood of PBB-exposed farm people when compared to controls. There was no correlation, however, between PBB concentrations in blood and lymphocyte number or level of lymphocyte function among samples obtained from Michigan farmers. No link has been established between these immunologic laboratory findings and the health of the people tested.

There is no doubt that the residents of dairy farms in Michigan have had more health complaints than their counterparts in other states [14–17]. No study, however, has shown a clear relationship between the blood or tissue levels of PBB in humans and the prevalence of severity of symptoms. All such studies are compounded by problems associated with the psychological impact on the farm families of the economic disaster coincident with the PBB accident.

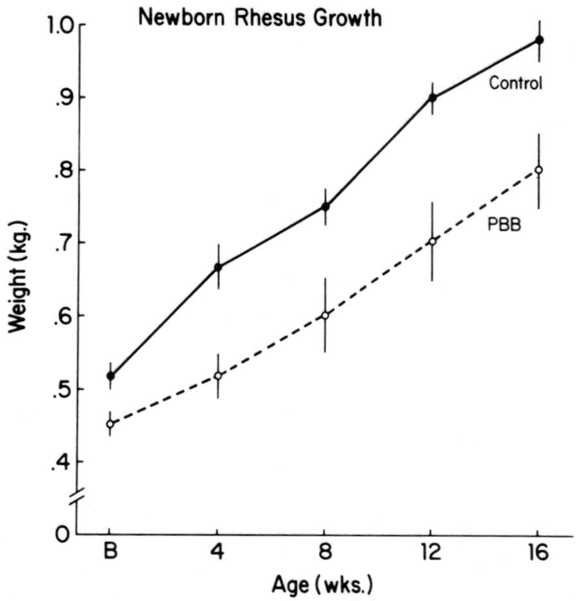

Fig. 1. Growth of newborn rhesus monkeys after prenatal and postnatal exposure to low levels of PBB (modified from data of Allen [12]).

Seagull [18] reports that certain skills measured by the McCarthy achievement scales for children were significantly depressed in 10 children with relatively high (above 0.1 ppm) blood levels of PBB when compared with nine children with lower levels. Barr [19] reported that the children with the highest PBB levels in his study had fewer illnesses and better school performance than matched children with lower PBB levels.

Reports on the half-life of PBB in man have also been in conflict. Isbister [20] reported a half-life in man between 10 and 11 months. Others have reported essentially no fall in tissue levels of PBB in man over 5 months [21] and over 2 years (Barr, personal communication). Lactating women excrete PBB faster than others.

The weight of evidence about the effects of PBB is growing. To date, no information has been collected to indicate that PBB is a teratogen or a carcinogen. Although the scientists and clinicians on the 1976 advisory panel did their best to devise a reasonable approach to the question of nursing with PBB-contaminated breast milk, we have a long way to go before we learn the true impact, if any, of that advice.

REFERENCES

1. Dunckel AE: An updating of the polybrominated biphenyl disaster in Michigan. JAVMA 167:838, 1975.
2. Kay K: Polybrominated biphenyls (PBB) environmental contamination in Michigan, 1973–1976. 13:74, 1977.

3. Jackson TF, Halbert F: A toxic syndrome associated with the feeding of polybrominated biphyl-contaminated protein concentrate to dairy cattle. JAVMA 165:437, 1974.
4. Willett LB, Irving HA: Distribution and clearance of polybrominated biphenyls by cows. J Dairy Sci 58:764, 1975.
5. Lillie RJ, Cecil HC, Bitman J, Fries CF: Toxicity of certain polychlorinated and polybrominated biphenyls on reproductive efficiency of caged chickens. Poultry Sci 54: 1500, 1975.
6. PBB Scientific Advisory Panel: Report to William G. Milliken, Governor of Michigan, on polybrominated biphenyls (PBB), May 24, 1976.
7. Sleight SD, Sanger VL: Pathologic features of polybrominated biphenyltoxicosis in the rat and guinea pig. JAVMA 169:1231, 1976.
8. Corbett TH, Beaudoin AR, Cornell RG, etal: Toxicity of polybrominated biphenyls (Firemaster BP-6) in rodents. Environ Res 10:390, 1975.
9. The Contamination Crisis in Michigan: Polybrominated Biphenyls. A report from the (Michigan) Senate Investigation Committee. July, 1975.
10. Gutenman WH, Lisk DJ: Tissue storage and excretion in milk of polybrominated biphenyls in ruminants. J Ag Food Chem 23:1005, 1975.
11. Fries GF, Marrow GS: Excretion of polybrominated biphenyls into the milk of cows. J Dairy Sci 58:947, 1975.
12. Allen JR, Lambrecht LK, Barsotti DA: Effects of polybrominated biphenyls in nonhuman primates. JAVMA 173:1485, 1978.
13. Bekesi JG, Holland JF, Anderson HA, et al: Lymphocyte function of Michigan dairy farmers exposed to polybrominated biphenyls. Science 199:1207, 1978.
14. Lilis R, Anderson HA, Valciukas JA, et al: Comparison of findings among residents on Michigan dairy farms and consumers of produce purchased from these farms. Environ Health Perspect 23:105 1978.
15. Valciukas JA, Lilis R, Wolf MS, Anderson HA: Comparative neurobehavioral study of a polybrominated biphenyl-exposed population in Michigan and a nonexposed group in Wisconsin. Environ Health Perspect 23:199, 1978.
16. Anderson HA, Lilis R, Selikoff IJ, et al: Unanticipated prevalence of symptoms among dairy farmers in Michigan and Wisconsin. Environ Health Perspect 23L217, 1978.
17. Barr M Jr: Pediatrics health aspects of PBB's. Environ Health Perspect 23:291, 1978.
18. Seagull EA: Developmental abilities of children exposed to polybrominated biphenyls. Press release from the Michigan Department of Public Health, Lansing, Michigan September 14, 1978.
19. Barr M: The paradox of PBB and Pediatric Patients. Abstract #34 in Annual Meeting of Midwest Society for Pediatric Research, Chicago, Illinois, November, 1978.
20. Isbister JL: PBB's in human health. Clin Med 84:22, 1977.
21. Humphrey HEB, Hayner NS: Polybrominated biphenyls: An agricultural incident and its consequences. II. An epidemiological investigation of human exposure. Trace Subst Environ Health 9:57, 1975.

Hormones and Related Substances in Milk

Alfred M. Bongiovanni, MD

The task assigned me is not an easy one. The metabolism excretion or secretion of drugs, hormones, and other substances in the maternal organism into milk has not enjoyed the thorough and almost religious scrutiny that has been the case with the kidney. Generally speaking, almost anything present in serum may be expected to be present in the milk, but the factors that govern these events, substance by substance, are not well understood. Certain elements, such as iodide, are actively concentrated in breast milk, as with the thyroid and salivary glands. The composition of milk varies with the stages of gestation and of various postpartum intervals. In particular the high fat content of colostrum diminishes almost daily after birth. This probably affects the excretion of lipid-soluble compounds. Milk is more acidic than serum and therefore tends to concentrate basic compounds. These are only a few considerations that determine the excretion of compounds in milk, and in the case of hormones very little is known. There are more questions than answers. Does the breast synthesize on its own certain hormones? Does it conjugate them into such compounds that elude standard methods of measurement? Apparently so. Does it metabolize them into unknown compounds that may nonetheless retain biological activity?

This review will attempt to outline what information is available on the presence of hormones in milk. It will include some limited discussion of other exogenous compounds excreted in milk, which affect certain endocrine glands. It will describe, where possible, likely effects on the suckling infant or the older child ingesting milk. Many studies to date are superficial and vague. All too often studies have only followed the course of administered radioactive hormones, and then only crude "counts" have been offered as data.

Drug and Chemical Risks to the Fetus and Newborn: 139–152

THYROID HORMONES

As a result of the observations of Tenore and associates [1] that breast-fed infants with cretinism fare better than those artificially nourished, there has been a recent outbreak of interest concerning thyroid hormones in human milk. In summary, by way of retrospective study, it was found that infants with congenital hypothyroidism who had been breast fed grew significantly better, exhibited more skeletal maturation and general development, and had better intellectual development. This improved performance in these several areas was noted to cease when infants were removed from the breast. In this same study, thyroxine was reported to be present in human milk.

It has been known for some years that aside from the thyroid gland, iodide is also concentrated by salivary and gastric glands as well as the mammae. It appears that only the last contains a peroxidase that will convert iodide to iodine, and this can be incorporated into certain proteins, but there is no evidence that the mammae per se can completely synthesize thyroid hormones. Man and Benotti [2] in 1969 reported large amounts of inorganic iodide in human milk but very little butanol extractable iodine.

With the advent of radioimmunoassay it has become possible to measure thyroid hormones in milk more accurately. In various publications to date, the quantities are not uniform, and there is a tendency for change depending on the time after gestation that the samples are collected. As yet there is little information on the relationship between the amount of hormone and the composition of the milk with respect to such items as fat or protein.

In 1976 Montalvo et al [3] studied human and simian milk samples. In four humans he found very little thyroxine immediately after birth, but this rose at one week to 9.6 μg/dl and fell thereafter. In monkeys there was consistently more, and the amount appeared adequate to protect the newborn from deficiency in the face of athyreosis. A year later a more extensive study appeared (Tenore et al [1]) showing an average of 5.4 μg thyroxine per dl at one month postpartum, 4.0 during the second month, 1.6 in the third, and 1.3 in the fourth. These investigators present evidence that even these small amounts seem to protect the athyrotic infant in a retrospective study of a large series.

Sack et al [4] found low thyroxine values in the first few days postpartum, rising to levels in the vicinity of 4.3 μg/dl between eight and 48 days but falling by 50 days to around 1 μg. These observers suggest that this quantity is enough to delay the recognition of the disorder in affected infants but in the long run is insufficient to prevent detrimental effects. They feel that any alleviation of the disease itself is of short duration. They also raise an interesting speculation. Does suckling, through the release of thyrotropin stimulating hormone (TRH), influence the secretion of both thyroid stimulating hormone TSH and prolactin? And may this influence the thyroid hormone content of the milk? Varma et al [5] measured several thyroid hormones in human milk. Thyroxine was below the limits of sensi-

TABLE I. Reported Concentrations of Thyroxine (T-4) and Triiodothyronine (T-3) in Human Milk at Various Times After Delivery

Age	T–4 (μg %)	T-3 (ng %)	Reference
1–4 weeks	5.4		Tenore, 1977 [1]
1–2 months	4.0		Tenore
2–4 months	1.6		Tenore
4–6 months	1.3		Tenore
3–7 days	0.8–1.3	133	Varma et al, 1978 [5]
96–128 days	0.7–1.4	136–286	Bode et al, 1978 [6]
1–7 weeks	4.3		Sack et al, 1977 [4]

tivity in some samples, but in most ranged between 0.8 and 1.3 μg/dl. Triiodothyronine displayed a broad range, was often zero in the first few days, but after day 8 postpartum reached 133 ng/dl; in many, however, it was not detectable. Their studies of reverse triiodothyronine revealed no significant correlation with the other levels. Bode and co-workers [6] measured thyroxine and triiodothyronine in the milk of five women between 96 and 128 days postpartum, and these results, with the others cited, are shown in Table I. In this last citation the authors also report one athyrotic infant who grew normally for ten months while he was breast fed, although the bone age was retarded. Growth decelerated with cessation of breast feeding. This single observation is interesting in light of the large series of Tenore et al [1]. These various findings are shown in Table I.

GOITROGENS

Many substances that interfere with the biosynthesis of thyroid hormones may be excreted into milk [8–10]. One of the most fascinating tales of contemporary medical history concerns the occurrence of seasonal endemic goiter in Tasmania during the 1950s. These endemics in school children were noted to coincide with the spring flush of the pastures. Its source was traced to wild turnips (family Brassicae) consumed by the cows in the pasture. These plants contain thioglucosides which release thiocyanates by hydrolysis of specific enzymes. Like the iodides, thiocyanates are concentrated in milk, and they inhibit both the uptake of iodine and its organification. This goiter is not relieved by iodide supplementation. The thioglucoside content of these plants, which include cabbage, kale, brussel sprouts and others, depends on the nature of the soil and the mode of cooking. These interesting events described in Tasmania [7, 8] have also been noted in Finland [9, 10]. Whether a similar problem might arise from human milk depending upon the maternal diet cannot at present be ascertained but is worth consideration.

It has long been known that medicinal antithyroid agents are secreted in milk. In 1944 Williams [11] reported levels of thiouracil in human milk which were three to 12 times those in the serum. A recent study by Low et al [12] concerns two infants whose mothers had been taking carbimazole, and both failed to show the expected surge in serum thyroxine at 24 hours of age; this probably is due to transplacental exposure, and nothing is said of the milk. However, it is clear that women who are taking any of this family of medications should not feed their infants at the breast. However, this writer has been unable to find any fully detailed report of the long-term consequences in such exposed infants. It is well known that the ingestion of iodides during pregnancy often produces goiter in the infant, as in the two cases reported by Martin and Rento [13]. Both babies had some evidence of temporary hypothyroidism. Since iodides are highly concentrated in milk, these should also be avoided during the period of breast feeding. The list of goitrogenic drugs is a long one, but there is little information on the concentration in milk and the effects in the nursling. Certainly the development of a goiter or hypothyroidism during infancy requires a thorough history of the maternal diet and medications as well as the usual studies recommended for these conditions.

VITAMIN D

Vitamin D is now regarded as a prohormone. For some years the matter of vitamin D in milk has been of interest. In general, breast-fed infants seem less susceptible to rickets than those artificially fed, but the matter is not entirely clear. There are sufficient reports of vitamin D deficiency in human breast-fed infants to raise questions. The literature, which will not be reviewed here, infrequently examines in meticulous detail the maternal state of nutrition, and the methods for analysis of the vitamin D content of maternal fluids are too recent to expect precise correlations. Hopefully, these will be forthcoming. Some data are shown in Table II.

Hartman and Dryden [14] found by bioassay 12 IU per liter vitamin D in human milk, but of course this can be extremely variable. Fresh cow's milk has been reported to contain 14 IU/liter in winter and 33 in summer [15]. The daily

TABLE II. Concentrations of Vitamin D in Human Milk

	IU per liter		
Human[a]	22		Macy and Kelly, 1961 [47] Hartman, 1965 [14]
Cow[a]	14 (winter)	33 (summer)	Watt and Merrill, 1963 [15]
Human[b]	400+		Lakdawala and Widdowson, 1977 [19]

[a]Bioassay.
[b]Colorimetric, including water soluble (sulfates).

requirement in infancy is probably 100–200 IU per day, although the daily recommended amount is 400 IU. Whether elevated quantities of vitamin D in the human mother may cause problems is virtually unknown. More is said of this possibility below. In 1972 [16] it was reported that a woman with hypoparathyroidism taking 50,000 IU of vitamin D daily had large amounts in her breast milk. This was present as 25-OH D, and her infant had modest hypercalcemia as well as cardiac anomalies, which did not, however, include supravalvular aortic stenosis. Kumar et al [17] found elevated values of 1,25-dihydroxy D in the plasm of pregnant women which rose with the length of gestation, and it remained elevated postpartum in those who continued to lactate. This occurred without any change in intake of the vitamin. Does pregnancy and lactation increase the critical hydroxylations of vitamin D? Almost nothing is known of these events, and we continue to depend on arbitrary recommendations for vitamin D supplements for infants. This matter requires further consideration and interpolation with many other events.

Perhaps the most confusing issue has arisen from the work of Sahashi who has reported the presence of vitamin D conjugates (sulfates) in human milk which are probably unaccounted for in the usual methods without prior hydrolysis. This conjugate is water soluble and escapes detection by the usual methods of the extraction of milk for the measurement of this vitamin by whatever method, and it has been isolated from both human and cow's milk. The sulfate in cow's milk is reported as 204 IU/liter and in human milk 950 IU. The administration of the conjugate to rabbits by mouth results in the urinary excretion of significant amounts. The important work cited here has been succinctly reviewed [18].

Lakdawala and Widdowson [19] found water-soluble vitamin D in human milk and in cow's milk as well. The amounts are considerable. Unfortunately, in these studies they employed a colorimetric technique (antimony chloride) rather than radioimmunoassay. However, this group is actively working on the explication of this matter. Therefore, human milk contains more vitamin D than had been earlier supposed, and the quantity in these studies approaches those in fortified artificial formulas. In the rat, vitamin D is sulfated in the liver. More details are needed about the activity of this conjugate and the relationship to the maternal status. No general conclusions can be drawn at this time, but this matter is an important one requiring further consideration.

The ingestion of certain plants by grazing cattle causes calcinosis and a clinical picture of hypervitaminosis D. There is hypercalcemia, hypophosphatemia, extensive soft tissue calcification, emaciation, and death. One plant that has been examined is Solanum malacoxylon [20]. Its extracts contain large amounts of a compound with the properties of 1,25-dihydroxy vitamin D, and it appears to be a close analogue of this active metabolite that does not require further activation. It is water soluble and can be hydrolyzed into a lipid-soluble substance by beta-glucosidase. The product of hydrolysis binds to the intestinal receptor for authentic 1,25-dihydroxy vitamin D [21]. Does this substance find its way into the milk? I cannot find the answer. Is this a possible source of the occasional mysterious iodiopathic hypercalcemia of infancy? Is it in fact confined to cow's milk and possibly artificial cow's milk formulae? Are there other plants containing this substance that are, at times and certain places, consumed by lactating women? These are matters of great concern in infant nutrition. It certainly does not come down to simplistic solutions such as specific recommendations for supplementation of infant feedings. One must know better what the mother or the cow is up to and whether these compounds are excreted in milk and absorbed by infants. Furthermore, vitamin D3 is now regarded as a prohormone, and as of this writing there is little or no information on the more active hydroxylated metabolites except under the unusual circumstances just described.

CORTICOIDS

Since glucocorticoids may be administered for appropriate reasons to nursing women, it is well to have some information on the concentrations in milk. However, because very serious maternal diseases requiring such treatment probably preclude nursing, the question may be academic. There is little information on this matter.

Using colorimetric methods, in 1956 Oka et al [22] reported baseline levels of free corticoids in human milk as 0–2.6 μg/dl. Following an intramuscular injection of 100 mg of either cortisone acetate or hydrocortisone acetate, the highest value obtained was 4.7 μg/dl at six hours. No glucuronide conjugates were found. These data are shown in Table III. In a single experiment Katz and Duncan [23] found in human milk 0.16 μg/dl prednisolone and 2.67 μg/dl prednisone two hours after a single oral dose of 10 mg prednisone. They regard these amounts as harmless to an infant. McKenzie et al [24] administered 5 mg of radioactive prednisolone to a single subject and found that 0.14% of the tag was secreted in milk during the

TABLE III. Range of Levels of Porter-Silber Chromogens (PS) in Human Milk, Baseline and at Various Times After Intramuscular Injection of Cortisone Acetate or Hydrocortisone Acetate

Free levels time	(PS chromogens – 8 women) μg %
0	0–2.6
6 hours	2.2–4.7
24 hours	1.5–3.0
Conjugates	Too low to measure

From Oka et al, 1956 [22].

subsequent 60 hours. They, too, believe the quantity to be negligible. In 1955 Mercier-Parot [25] reported growth retardation and death in rat sucklings whose mothers had been given 20 mg cortisone acetate by mouth daily. Admittedly, this is a very large dose, but it must be concluded that the issue is not settled.

PREGNANEDIOL

In 1964 Arias and associates [26] found that the milk of women whose infants became jaundiced contained 3α,20β-pregnanediol. Thus for some years this steroid has been thought culpable, especially since it had been shown to inhibit glucuronide conjugation by rat liver in vitro. Furthermore, these workers [27] produced hyperbilirubinemia in two healthy newborn infants by feeding this compound. More recently this issue has been questioned. Not all workers have succeeded in isolating this steroid under such circumstances, and Adlard and Lathe were unable to demonstrate any such inhibition employing human liver slices [28]. Hargreaves and Piper [29] do not believe that this steroid is the sole factor in producing hyperbilirubinemia. The source of this steroid in human milk is not known, although it must be presumed to originate from the gonads or the adrenal cortices. In clinical practice these findings have often led to the prohibition of continued breast feeding. There are still many unanswered questions on this issue. Probably several factors are involved, and usually the condition is not so severe as to contraindicate breast feeding. Surely, there are instances of unexplained hyperbilirubinemia that do not involve factors in breast milk. Further investigation is merited.

SEX HORMONES

The matter of the possible presence of sex steroids in milk derived from various formulations for ovulation control in human milk is important, but the significance is not known, and the studies are few and often sketchy. Although breast feeding has a contraceptive effect, this is variable and not reliable. Thus, it would be surprising if many nursing mothers were not taking oral contraceptives to avoid an early subsequent pregnancy.

In general such observations as are available show only a minute fraction of these hormones in human milk, but there are questions. For example, the possibility of undetected conjugates has not been thoroughly answered. The free hormones are likely to be present in larger quantities in the fatty milk of the early postnatal period and the post-nursing milk, and there may be some relation between the concentration of such steroids in milk and the concentration of sex hormone binding porteins.

At present there is no evidence of significant side-effects in human infants [30], but there are rare reports of gynecomastia in nursing infants [31]. There are far more anecdotal occurrences among those of us who practice pediatric endocrinology, but solid facts are few. It does appear that the incidence of infantile gynecomastia in several clinics has increased since the introduction of "the pill" in the mid-1950s, but nothing more can reliably be said on this issue. There have been no noteworthy effects in monkeys, and in rats there has been no effect on later life, including reproduction. These matters have recently been summarized [30].

There is some older literature on the appearance of sex steroids in the milk of experimental animals. In 1930 Courier [32] administered "estrin" to nursing guinea pigs, and within three to four days the sucklings showed vaginal opening. Lacassagne [33] found estrogenic activity in human colostrum, 0.5 ml of which produced cornification of the vagina in spayed mice when administered subcutaneously. Although there is little information on androgens, in 1938 Raynaud [34] found that when such was administered to lactating animals, it was excreted in milk. All of these studies employed bioassay.

There have been a number of studies measuring the excretion of radioactively labeled compounds in the milk. Most of these are difficult to interpret. The exact nature or biological activity of the substances measured is unknown, and attempts to derive quantitative information are questionable. In 1966 Pincus and his colleagues [35] found that 19-norsteroids were excreted in milk by such methods, but they reported that no estrogenic activity was present. Laumas and his group, who have contributed greatly in this area [36] found 0.45–1.52% of administered tagged norethyndrol over the next five days' collection of milk. This compound is 17α-ethynyl-17β-hydroxy-oestr-5(10)-en-3-one and was administered orally as the 5 mg tablet of Enovid. Two days of pretreatment with this drug, untagged, was practiced in these studies. The biological activity of the excreted label is unknown. Van der Molen [37] studied orally administered 19-nor-17α-ethinyl-testosterone, 5 mg/day. He studied excretion in urine and milk. The latter contained 0.022–0.088% of the label. Based on an intake of 600 ml milk daily by the infant, it is calculated that 8 μg of the compound are ingested. Not all such calculations will be summarized here since there is some disagreement among workers on the quantity excreted and the mathematical devices employed. Here, too, the biological activity of the products is unknown, but the authors cite the work of Lauritzen in 1967 showing the estrogenization of the vagina in infants feeding from mothers on oral contraceptives. As an extension of earlier studies on norethyndrol, Laumas [38] reports biologic estrogenic activity in the milk of two of three women studied. This worker also found that 0.124–0.485% of radioactivity was excreted in milk after the oral administration of 6-chloro-6-dehydro-17α-acetoxyprogesterone [39].

There are now studies employing radioimmunoassay, but here, too, it must be emphasized that, despite the specificity of these techniques, there is no information on metabolites of the administered steroids that may or may not be biologically active. In 1975 Baghat and co-workers [40] studied the excretion of progestins (Gestagen R2323) implanted into rhesus monkeys. The animals were followed for 12 weeks; in the early part of the experiment the blood/milk ratio was almost 1.0, whereas later it was closer to 2.0. These workers calculated that a nursling would ingest 0.3 μg of the compound daily when the maternal blood level was 1–2 ng/ml, which is a contraceptive level. An extremely detailed study has been carried out by Saxena [41], and these data have been transcribed into diagrams shown in Figures 1 and 2. Seven lactating women were given 150 mg intramuscular medroxyprogesterone acetate (MPA) one week after delivery. Milk and maternal plasma levels fell very slowly and were similar up to 87 days of study (see Fig. 1). Five women took orally 350 μg 17α-ethinyl-19-nor-testosterone (NET), and levels were followed for 24 hours (Fig. 2). The levels in milk were one-tenth those of maternal plasma. Limited studies in two women who were given 30 μg ethinylestradiol plus 150 μg of 13β-ethyl-17α-ethinyl testosterone were performed on days 6 and 12, and only the progestin was measured. The levels in milk were 135–180 pg/ml, about one-twentieth those of the maternal plasma. Nilsson et al [42] studied three groups two months after delivery while

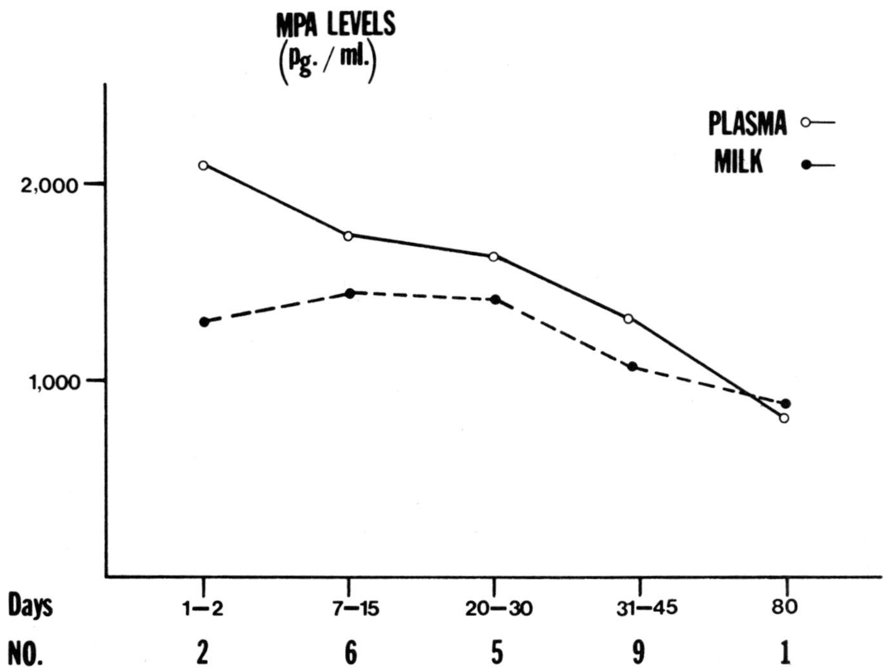

Fig. 1. Levels (average of seven subjects) of medroxyprogesterone in maternal plasma and milk after a single injection of cortisone acetate, 150 mg Im. These data have been extrapolated from Saxena et al [41].

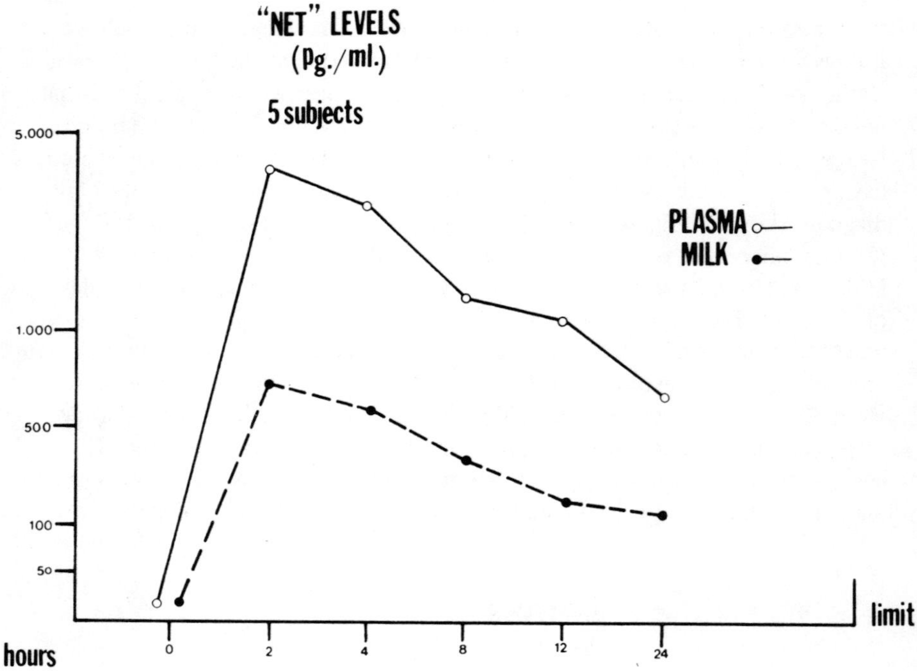

Fig. 2. Plasma and milk levels of 17-ethinyl-19-nor testosterone after an oral dose of 350 μg. The average of five subjects is shown and has been extrapolated from the data of Saxena et al [41].

taking oral contraceptives. All were given 13β-ethyl-17α-ethinyl testosterone in doses of 30 μg, 150 μg, or 250 μg. The second group was given 30 μg and the third 50 μg of estradiol as well. Only the progestin was measured, and there was none in the milk of the first group. In the second and third groups the milk levels were 0.17–0.54 and 0.38–1.05 ng/ml, respectively. The plasma levels of two infants in the third group were very low or zero.

If some contraceptive agents in some parts of the world continue to include estrogens, more studies need to be done on this group of steroids, and more detailed information is needed on the metabolism of all steroids that appear in milk. It is really difficult to draw any firm conclusions of clinical significance from this conglomeration of information.

MISCELLANEOUS

There are a few single reports of other hormones found in human milk. Osud [43] reports small amounts of corticotropin, epinephrine, and insulin, none of

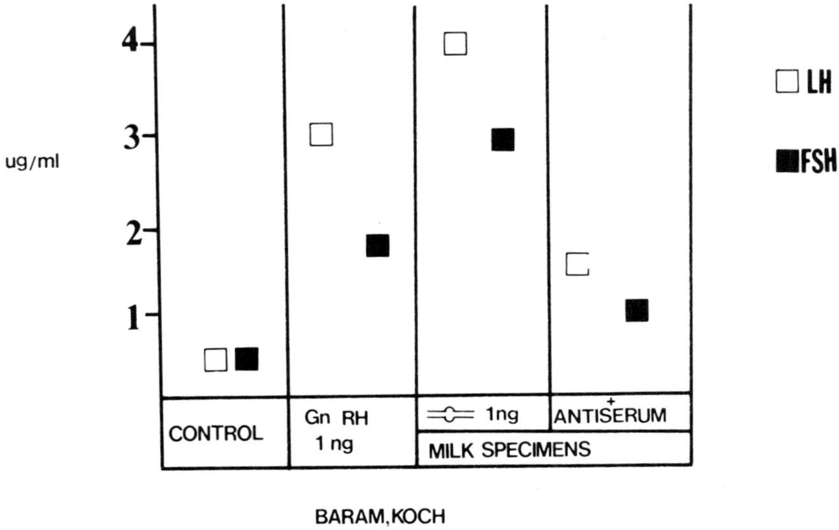

Fig. 3. Effect of extract of 4.5 liters of cow's milk on release of luteinizing (LH) and follicle stimulating (FSH) hormones into medium from 12-day-old male rat pituitaries in vitro. Data have been interpolated from Baram et al [45]. Right-hand column shows neutralization of milk extract by specific antiserum.

which appear significant. Oxytocin administered to the mother may also be secreted into the milk. By the techniques of radioimmunoassay it is reported by Gala et al [44] that prolactin is present in human milk and that its levels correlate directly with those in serum, but the amounts are small.

Baram et al [45] have found gonadotropin releasing hormone (GnRH) in cow's milk. After suitable extraction the amounts were measured by radioimmunoassay and bioassay through the effects on rat pituitaries in vitro. The data of these workers on the bioassay of the releasing hormone in milk has been translated into Figure 3. As shown therein the levels of activity were suppressed if the milk extract was treated with specific antibody against GnRH. It was calculated that the results correspond to 1.5 ng of GnRH per milliliter of milk. The work of Forest et al [46] has shown a rise in serum testosterone and gonadotropins during the first few months of life in human male infants. Baram [45] finds that the rise in luteinizing hormone in newborn rats is prevented if they are denied their mother's milk. Does then GnRH in breast milk explain these interesting hormonal events of the first few months of life? Might it also not explain the "masculinization" of the hypothalamus in males whose testes are stimulated in early infancy by GnRH in milk? These are crucial questions and point to yet another if rather unexpected argument in favor of breast feeding. There has not been to date a deluge of clinical reports concerning such expected malfunction in those fed nutriments other than milk. Nonetheless, there is room for further study. Baram [45] also reports very small amounts of TRH in cow's milk.

DISCUSSION

It is apparent that the information on the uptake, metabolism, and secretion/excretion of hormones by the mammae is incomplete. Some aspects of the problem represent potential threats to the suckling infant. Probably the most widely employed hormones that do find their way into milk are those used for contraception. Available studies seem to show little if any detrimental effect despite the intake of such agents at a low level by infants, but the matter requires further study and suggests advantages to very low dose programs. On the other hand, may there be "normally" transmitted hormones from mother to infant which play a role in development? This may be the case, as with the gonadotropin releasing hormones. At present there are more questions than answers, and the field is open to additional study.

REFERENCES

1. Tenore A, Parks JS, Bongiovanni AM: In Chiumello G, Laron Z (eds): "Relationship of Breast Feeding to Congenital Hypothyroidism." Rec Prog Ped Endocr, Proc Serono Symposia. London: Academic Press 1977, p 213–230.
2. Man EB, Benotti J: Butanol extractable iodine in human and bovine milk. Clin Chem 15:1141, 1969.
3. Montalvo JM, Wahner HW, Christie RJ: Triiodothyronine and Thyroxine Levels in the Milk of Humans and Primates. Prog, 56th Meeting, American Endocrine Society, 1976, p A-91.
4. Sack J, Amado O, Lunenfeld B: Thyroxine concentration in human milk. J Clin Endocrinol Metab 45:171, 1977.
5. Varma SK, Collins M, Haller WS, Varma K: Thyroxine, T3 and reverse T3 in human milk. J Pediatr 93:803, 1978.
6. Bode HH, Vanjonack WJ, Crawford JD: Mitigation of cretinism by breast feeding. Pediatrics 62:13, 1978.
7. Clements WF, Wischart JW: A thyroid blocking agent in the etiology of endemic goiter. Metabolism 5:623, 1956.
8. Gibson HB, Howeler JF, Clements FW: Seasonal epidemics of endemic goiter in Tasmania. Med J Aust 1:875, 1960.
9. Petola P, Krusins FE: Effect of Cow's milk from the goiter endemic district of Finland on thyroid function. Acta Endocrinol (Kbh) 33:603, 1960.
10. Arstila A, Krusins FE, Petola P: Studies on the transfer of thio-oxazolidone type goitrogens into cow's milk. Acta Endocrinol (Kbh) 60:712, 1969.

11. Williams RH, Kay GH, Jandorf BF: Thiouracil: Its absorption, distribution and excretion. J Clin Invest 23:613, 1944.
12. Low LCK, Ratcliffe WA, Alexander WD: Intrauterine hypothyroidism due to anti-thyroid drug therapy during pregnancy. Lancet 2:370, 1978.
13. Martin MM, Rento RD: Iodide goiter with hypothyroidism in two newborn infants. J Pediatr 61:94, 1962.
14. Hartman AM, Dryden LP: Vitamins in Milk and Milk Products. American Dairy Science Association, 1965.
15. Watt BK, Merrill EL: Cited in Fomon SJ (ed): "Infant Nutrition," Ed 2. Philadelphia: WB Saunders, 1974.
16. Goldberg LD: Transmission of a vitamin D metabolite in breast milk. Lancet 2:1258, 1972.
17. Kumar R, Cohen WR, Silva P, Epstein FH: Elevated 1,25-dihydroxy-vitamin D in normal human pregnancy. J Clin Invest 63:342, 1979.
18. Editorial: Vitamin D sulfate. Nutr Rev 28:73, 1970.
19. Lakdawala DR, Widdowson EM: Vitamin D in human milk. Lancet 1:167, 1977.
20. Wasserman RH, Henion JD, Haussler MR, McCain TA: Calcinogenic factor in solanum malcoxylone. Science 194:853, 1976.
21. Editorial: 1,25-Dihydroxycholecalciferol from a plant. Lancet 1:233, 1977.
22. Oka M, Wasz-Hockert O, Widholm O: 17-Hydroxyprogesterone in human milk. Experientia 11:426, 1956.
23. Katz FH, Duncan BR: Entry of prednisone into human milk. N Engl J Med 293:1154, 1975.
24. McKenzie SA, Selley JA, Agnew JE: Secretion of prednisone into breast milk. Obstet Gynecol Surv 31:529, 1976.
25. Mercier-Parot L: Disturbance in postnatal development of rats after maternal administration of cortisone. Comp Rend 240:2259, 1955.
26. Arias IM, Gartner LM, Seifter S, Furman M: Prolonged neonatal unconjugated hyperbilirubinemia associated with breast feeding. J Clin Invest 43:2037, 1964.
27. Arias IM, Gartner LM: Production of hyperbilirubinemia in full term infants following administration of 3α, 20β-pregnanediol. Nature 203:1292, 1964.
28. Adlard BPF, Lathe GH: Breast milk jaundice. Arch Dis Child 45:186, 1970.
29. Hargreaves T, Piper R: Breast milk jaundice. Arch Dis Child 45:186, 1970.
30. Nilsson S, Nygren K: Transfer of contraceptive steroids to human milk. Res Reprod 11:1, 1979.
31. Curtis EM: Oral contraceptive feminization of a normal male infant. Obstet Gynecol 23:295, 1964.
32. Courier R: Cited in Burrows E, "Biological Actions of Sex Hormones," Ed 2. Cambridge University Press, 1949, p 352.
33. Lacassagne A, Nyka W: Ibid, p 318.
34. Raynaud A: Ibid, p 192.
35. Pincus G, Bialy G, Layne DS, Paniugua MP, Williams KI: Radioactivity in the milk of subjects receiving 19-norsteroids. Nature 212:924, 1966.
36. Laumas KR, Malkani PK, Bhatnagar S, Laumas V: Radioactivity in breast milk after oral administration on ^{3}H-norethyndrel. Am J Obstet Gynecol 98:411, 1967.
37. Van der Molen HJ, Hart PG, Wijmeriga HG: Studies with 4-^{14}C-lynestrenol in Normal and Lactating Women. Acta Endocrinol (Kbh) 61:255, 1969.
38. Laumas V, Malkani PK, Laumas KR: The possibility of estrogenic activity in the milk of lactating women after oral administration of gestogens. Contraception 2:331, 1970.
39. Laumas KR: Metabolism of Progestational Steroids in Women. Excerpta Med Internat. Congress Series #219:907, 1971.

40. Baghat M, Atkinson LE, Brunson AO, Segal SJ: Treatment of postpartum rhesus monkeys with progestins: Appearance in milk. Contraception 12:665, 1975.
41. Saxena BN, Shrimanker K, Grudzinskas JG: Levels of Contraceptive steroids in breast milk and plasma of lactating women. Contraception 16:605, 1977.
42. Nilsson S, Nygren K, Johansson EDB: Norgestel concentration in maternal plasma, milk and children's plasma during administration of oral contraceptives. Am J Obstet Gynecol 129:178, 1977.
43. Osud BJ: Breast feeding and infant health. Clin Obstet Gynecol 18:149, 1975.
44. Gala RR, Singhakowinta A, Brennan MJ: Studies on prolactin in human serum, urine and milk. Hormone Res 6:310, 1975.
45. Baram T, Koch Y, Hazum E, Fridkin M: Gonadotropins releasing hormone in milk. Science 198:300, 1977.
46. Forest MG, Sizonenko PL, Cathiard AM, Bertrand J: Hypophysogonadal function in humans during the first year of life. J Clin Invest 53:819, 1974.
47. Macy IG, Kelly HJ: in Fomon SJ (ed): "Infant Nutrition," Ed. 2, Philadelphia: W.B. Saunders, 1974.

The Obstetrician's View

Richard H. Schwarz, MD

The classic measures of the quality of obstetric and neonatal care have been for many years maternal and perinatal mortality. Both have been steadily reduced over the years and perhaps in the foreseeable future will reach an irreducible minimum. It is obviously insufficient, however, to view the problem in such a crude manner. Indeed, even assessment of perinatal morbidity has generally been limited to the presence or absence of gross abnormalities present at birth or detected in early infancy. It would seem clear, however, that mortality and gross morbidity are but the tip of the iceberg and that it is only with long-term physical, neurological, and behavioral follow-up that the quality of the reproductive product can be judged. The birth of a normal-appearing baby with good Apgar scores and a normal neonatal course, although encouraging and probably generally associated with a good long-term outlook, cannot be totally reassuring. In order then to evaluate the impact of drugs and chemical risks on the fetus and newborn, it seems apparent that one need is the development of more precise, reproducible, and comparable methods for making these assessments. It is not difficult to appreciate the impact of the maternal use of alcohol when the newborn evidences the entire spectrum of the fetal alcohol syndrome, but are there more subtle long-term effects in the phenotypically normal child?

A second concern and an especially important one for the obstetrician involves therapeutic drugs in pregnancy. One would have anticipated that the thalidomide-phocomelia story would have led to a significant reduction in drug use during pregnancy. This was, I believe, especially to be anticipated in view of the heightened interest on the part of consumers in noninterference and "natural" approaches to childbirth. In fact, however, it does not appear that the level of therapeutic drug exposure has been appreciably lessened. In one study, the number of drug exposures per patient during the course of pregnancy was five or more in 93% of patients. The list of drugs according to frequency of use is presented in Table I. As anticipated, vitamin and iron supplements are at the top,

Drug and Chemical Risks to the Fetus and Newborn: 153–156

TABLE I. Medication Consumption by Pregnant Women

Prenatal (n = 168)	% Patients receiving one or more drugs from each class
Iron	100.0
Analgesics	95.5
Vitamins	80.4
Topical ointments, suppositories, douches	72.0
Antacids	56.0
Topical anti-infectives	49.4
Cough and cold medicines	41.1
Miscellaneous	37.5
Laxatives	37.5
Antibiotic/anti-infective	36.9
Unknown medications	26.2
Antiemetics	19.0
Barbiturates	17.9
Antihistamines	17.9
Illicit drugs	13.1
Intravenous fluids	11.9
Hormones	6.5
Nonbarbiturate hypnotics	4.2
Nutritional supplements	4.2
Diuretics	2.4
Appetite suppressants	2.4

From Doering and Stewart: JAMA, 1978.

and although these are generally passed off as being both useful and innocuous, the evidence is not clear in supporting the need for vitamins in healthy women with reasonable diets; in addition, although the need for iron is more evident, its routine use may also be questioned. Many of the other drugs that are utilized frequently such as analgesics, antacids, sedatives, and tranquilizers are most frequently applied for the relief of symptoms rather than the treatment of a specific health or life threat. Physicians and patients alike should learn to resist the automatic response of a prescription for every symptom offered. Mild nausea and vomiting of early pregnancy may well be controlled by dietary modification, and even more severe forms requiring hospitalization can often be dealt with by bed rest and intravenous fluid and electrolyte replacement without the use of antiemetics. On the other hand, it is clearly not my intent to promote therapeutic nihilism. The decision to treat must always be based upon a balance between the need and the risks. Obviously the patient with acute pyelonephritis and a fever of 103°F requires treatment. The consequences to both the patient and her pregnancy are so serious that the balance is not in doubt. The problem in such a patient is not whether to treat but rather with which agent. It is then the responsibility of the physician to understand the antibiotics from which he will choose, not only from a perspective of their antimicrobial activity but also, in this special circumstance, to appreciate both maternal and fetal toxicity and the alterations in pharmacokinetics brought about by pregnancy.

Until rather recently the concerns of obstetricians and their patients were almost exclusively for those drugs and chemicals to which there was a known and voluntary exposure. More recently, however, there has emerged a rapidly expanding pool of information of varying quality concerning the potential, and in some cases actual, effects of environmental chemicals. These include food additives, industrial and occupational hazards, as well as environmental pollutants some of which are geographically specific. Exposure is in most cases not voluntary or if it is, not with a background of appropriate information. It is also evident epidemiologically that with most of these agents either the attack rate is low or the effects are subtle or long-term, otherwise they would be quickly related. The difficulties that are encountered by the clinician with regard to environmental chemical hazards are related in large part to the acquistion of information and to evaluation of the confusing, often conflicting, advice that he receives from multiple sources. One cannot help but conclude that in a great many instances the method of presentation of information and, indeed, the data themselves are skewed dramatically, depending upon the source and the vested interests of that source. There are certainly numerous examples, but suffice it to say that the views of the American Cancer Society and those of the Tobacco Industry spokesmen on the hazards of smoking do not coincide. The consumer and the clinician both need help in sorting out this confusion. The recent events at Three Mile Island, Pennsylvania, I believe provide a classic and quite dramatic example of our lack of well-documented information in this area. Although the dangers went far beyond those to the unborn child, the lack of uniform advice and policy was evident from the start. Well-meaning but variously informated individuals and groups at all levels offered information and recommendations, usually in quite an authoritative manner. These sources ranged from the individual citizen, to local, state or federal government, as well as all levels of the media. A variety of "experts" was trotted out to analyze the situation, often from a television studio 3,000 miles from the scene. The obvious problem, of course, was that even though many of these media experts were indeed quite well qualified from the standpoint of background knowledge and expertise, they were usually working in the specific case from a base of total ignorance of the real or potential radiation levels. Needless to say, the agencies in control of the situation walked on a tightrope between the creation of uncontrolled panic and the provision of appropriate information to the public.

But let us assume for the moment the very best; let us assume that engineers were able to give us precise information about the radiation level at the site and further let us assume that we were dealing with a totally stable situation in which the levels would remain, at least for the short term, constant. Would we be prepared to give precise recommendations to the population? Who should be evacuated? How far should they move? Do pregnant women need to move farther away? Is there a difference between those in the first trimester and those in later pregnancy? What about the lactating woman and her child? I submit to you that we are not prepared to answer these questions.

To be sure this is a dramatic illustration, but the message applies equally to other environmental hazards. The consumer is in need of information. The pregnant woman expects her physician to supply this information, but the physician may well be overwhelmed by the enormous volume of confusing and contradictory data. The challenge for the future, I believe, lies with the researchers. I believe that the emphasis should be on mechanisms whereby this damage is produced. Since human investigation is necessarily limited to retrospective analysis and epidemiologic study, the use of animal models is imperative. The translation of such data to the human is, however, fraught with difficulty unless it can be shown that mechanisms are common. In addition, researchers must continue in the area of evaluation and detection of the more subtle abnormalities as well as in the study of potential dangers of specific agents. Only with this kind of research can the obstetrician be provided with data that is free of the biases of interest groups, or even the overzealous consumer interests, and thereby have a basis for sound advice. The challenge then to the obstetrician will be to assimilate this information as provided and interpret it for the patient in a rational and sensitive fashion. Without this latter step, I fear we might well develop a population of patients who would fear eating, drinking water or milk or a glass of champagne on their wedding anniversary, indeed even breathing. The knowledge is essential; the perspective, imperative.

Summary: Pediatrician's View

Sumner J. Yaffe, MD

This symposium has clearly demonstrated that drugs and environmental chemicals may act upon the developing fetus and newborn infant and at times produce adverse effects. The developmental status of the immature host is a major determinant of the resultant drug action. Exposure may occur in utero with placental transmission of foreign compounds or through breast milk in the suckling infant. Irrespective of the route of administration, the immature organism will serve as a recipient of the medication that was prescribed for the treatment of maternal disease. Although transport mechanisms across the placenta or breast may be quite different and, indeed, remain to be delineated, it is quite clear, and unfortunate, that in neither instance does an effective filtration barrier exist. In fact, we should accept the generalization that all drugs administered to the mother will reach the fetus or suckling infant. There will be exceptions, of course, to this truism, and it is important that we recognize these, because knowledge of these exceptions may enable us to treat the maternal organism without fetal or neonatal exposure. For example, some drugs may be altered during transplacental passage or during their absorption from the gastrointestinal tract of the suckling infant. We can employ these drugs in treating maternal disease if we have this specific knowledge. Similarly, the extent of drug binding to plasma protein is important for us to consider because only the free, non-protein-bound drug will cross membranes, and we can use this information to advantage in treating disease in the mother or, conversely, in using the maternal route to treat fetal disease. In the latter case, one would use a drug with relatively little protein binding so as to permit as much drug as possible to reach the fetus.

As the final speaker I should like to focus attention on two concepts that have been developed during this symposium and to expand on these somewhat, because I think that they deserve additional emphasis. The first concerns appreciation of the fact that toxic manifestations of intrauterine exposure to environmental agents

Drug and Chemical Risks to the Fetus and Newborn: 157–161

may be subtle, quite unexpected, and also delayed. The second concerns the recent observation that drug exposure of the father may influence the outcome of pregnancy. Before discussing these two aspects I should like also to point out that while we have singled out and separated the obstetrician from the pediatrician for these summary statements, it is quite clear that this was done only for logistical purposes and that both specialties must work together to define the risks of drug and chemical exposure of the fetus and newborn infant.

Our concern for the delayed effects of drugs following intrauterine exposure was first raised following the tragic discovery that females exposed in utero to diethylstilbestrol (DES) had a high incidence of vaginal carcinoma. The malignancy was not discovered until after puberty. Thus 15–20 years were required for this effect of the intrauterine exposure to be noted. It has become apparent that the male offspring were also affected, and they have abnormalities of the reproductive system with epididymal cysts, hypotrophic testes, capsular induration, and pathologic semen. Ironically, the original purpose of the study, a reduction in the complications of pregnancy, showed that stilbesterol was no more effective than placebo. I should like to expand upon this concept of long-term latency and delayed effect by sharing some data with you regarding recent experiments that have been conducted in our laboratories by Drs. C. Gupta, B. Shapiro, and B. Sonawane. In these investigations they studied the widely used hypnotic-sedative agent phenobarbital. Phenobarbital is an old drug which is not only widely prescribed but is also a component of many multi-ingredient pharmaceutical preparations. It is quite clear that, like most agents, usage of this drug does not abate during pregnancy. Long-term consequences, particularly on the developing organism of intrauterine exposure, are not known. Dr. Gupta had shown in previous experiments that phenobarbital can act upon the neuroendocrine axis in adult animals to affect reproductive function. It therefore seemed appropriate to investigate the effects of phenobarbital exposure to the fetus and to correlate biologic changes observed with measurements of steroid sex hormones at various stages of postnatal development.

Timed-pregnant Sprague-Dawley rats were given 40 mg of phenobarbital per kilogram of body weight from day 12 to day 19 of gestation. The drug was administered subcutaneously once a day in the morning. This dose of phenobarbital is without noticeable affect upon the mother. Activity and function were normal. The pregnancy was uneventful, and the treated mothers delivered normal litters, both as far as malformations and the number of offspring were concerned. After birth, body weight of the offspring was recorded every five days until adulthood was reached. Eye opening (normal age, approximately 14 days) and startle and righting reflexes (normal appearance, 15–20 days) were examined in the offspring. Around 35 days, the onset of puberty normally takes place. This biologic event was determined by examining the time for vaginal opening and analyzing the vaginal smear. At several times during the life-cycle, animals were sacrificed, and reproductive organ weight was recorded, and hormone level and receptor level for the hormone were measured.

Some of the animals were allowed to develop to adults, and at that time their estrous cycle and fertility were examined. Again, at the time of sacrifice, reproductive organ weights and hormone and receptor levels were measured.

Since the growth rate of an animal in many instances is an important indicator of normal development, we recorded body weight for the duration of the experiment. The animals receiving phenobarbital in utero were significantly smaller than control animals, starting shortly before weaning and continuing to the end of the maximum growth spurt in adulthood. After plateau growth had been reached, there was no significant difference between the treated and the control animals.

Among the various biologic parameters examined, such as startle reflex, righting reflex, and eye opening, the first striking difference noticed was the first day of vaginal opening. There was a significant delay of two to three days in vaginal opening times in the females that were exposed to phenobarbital in utero. Vaginal opening time signifies the onset of puberty in the female rat. When these animals reached adulthood (approximately 60 days of age), vaginal smears were examined in order to determine whether these animals had a regular estrous cycle. The normal cycle is defined as two days of estrous (as determined by vaginal smear) followed by two to three days of diestrous. We found in the control group, as we expected, that 100% of the animals had a normal cycle, whereas only one-third of the treated animals had a normal cycle. Prolonged estrous was seen in about one-half of the phenobarbital-treated animals. This indicates that the animals had an abnormal cycle, since only on rare occasions would they go on to the diestrous phase. Twenty percent of the treated animals had a constant estrous and never went on to diestrous, as determined by vaginal smear. The fertility of the treated animals was determined by mating them with known fertile males. While 100% of control animals receiving saline while they were in utero were fertile, only 40% of those females that were exposed to phenobarbital were fertile. Another 40% of the treated animals resorbed their fetuses, as determined by examining the implantation size, and 20% of the treated animals could not conceive at all. Resorption or infertility were never seen in the control group. So far we do not know the mechanism or the molecular events involved in the reproductive dysfunction observed in the female rats that received phenobarbital in utero. We did examine circulating levels of sex hormones such as estrogen and progesterone, since reproductive function is usually correlated with these levels. We thought that it was important to know whether the circulating levels of these hormones were altered by phenobarbital exposure and whether this, in turn, was the cause of the defects in reproduction that we observed. We found that estrogen concentrations were higher before puberty and during adulthood in the treated animals. No difference, however, was noted on the day of vaginal opening. Progesterone concentrations were also higher before puberty, but the difference was no longer significant after puberty. Although circulating hormone levels are responsible for certain reproductive functions, action at the molecular level is mediated by combination with specific hormone receptors. We examined concentrations of these in the uterus and found that they were significantly higher at all periods of development. It is possible that the high levels of estrogen resulted in increased synthesis of receptor protein. Alternatively, the increased cytoplasmic receptor level may indicate either a defective conversion of cytoplasmic to nuclear receptor or a decrease in the permeability of the nucleus to the cytoplasmic receptor. It is also possible that the nuclear receptor is less responsive to the hormone and, as a consequence, higher amounts of hormone and cytosolic receptor were synthesized.

The clinical significance of these animal experiments is unknown, but the striking and permanent effects upon reproductive function warrant careful scrutiny of the safety of these agents during human pregnancy. Many other psychotrophic agents are taken by women during pregnancy. We are in the process of investigating these agents in laboratory animals. I would not be surprised if they also had long-term delayed effects upon biologic function in the offspring that are exposed at critical periods of development.

The other area I would like to highlight is the influence of drug exposure of the father on perinatal outcome. This is an area that has not received very much attention from the research community in contrast to the markedly increased research efforts concerning the effects of maternal drug ingestion – research stimulated by the thalidomide disaster several decades (!) ago. It should be mentioned that thalidomide itself, when given to male rabbits before breeding, results in significantly higher death rates among the offspring. Other compounds taken by the male are also capable of affecting the outcome of pregnancy. These include narcotics, such as morphine and methadone, to which many males are not regularly exposed. On the other hand they also include common substances such as ethanol, caffeine, and propoxyphene. In addition to these drugs, paternal exposure to lead will result in decreased litter size, birthweight, and survival. The mechanisms underlying the phenomenon of paternally mediated effects upon the progeny are unknown. It is likely that more than one mechanism is involved. The possibilities for these effects include damage to the male germ cells, as for example alteration in chromosome structure. Another possibility is that the drug or chemical is present in the seminal fluid, and this might alter sperm motility and function, or the drugs in the semen might have some influence on the uterus with consequent effects upon placentation, or the drugs in the semen might serve as a route of administration for systemic absorption in the maternal organism through the vaginal mucosa. It is quite clear that further research is needed to delineate the mechanisms accounting for the effects of paternally ingested drugs and chemicals. This research should not only elucidate the mechanisms for the effects but also determine the classes of drugs and chemicals that are capable of producing these effects. In addition, the duration of the effect must also be investigated. The clinical implications of these animal studies must remain speculative at present; nonetheless, it would seem to be advisable for practitioners to caution against the use of drugs around the time of coitus when pregnancy might result. In fact, in this era of planned parenthood the potential father must be made aware of the possibility of effects resulting from his intake of drugs and chemicals. The very possibility of adverse effects on the offspring might be used to motivate males to modify health-threatening behaviors, just as the possibility of pregnancy may motivate a potential mother to quit smoking or drinking, because of her concern for the infant.

These two examples have been cited in depth because they serve to compound the task of the preclinical assessment of safety. Obviously therapeutic nihilism (by the physician) is one solution to the safety problem. But, of course, this does not apply to medications that are purchased over the counter or to environmental agents. In many of these instances the subject does not even know of his or her exposure. Traditional animal tests are certainly not predictive and cannot be relied upon to supply answers. What is needed is an understanding of mechanisms at the molecular level, so that animal models can be developed which are rational and which can then be used in the reliable assessment of safety. Long-term effects in particular will not be elucidated in the human because the very nature of the period of observation is beyond the interest or ability of clinical investigators. Animals with a much shortened life-cycle are clearly of value, but modeling must be based upon science and not regulations promulgated by government. Finally, we must remember that fetal diagnosis is at hand, and fetal therapeutics will soon follow. We must develop sufficient data from human studies to make the administration of drugs to the fetus for the treatment of fetal disease as sound and rational as is therapeutics in the adult organism. This requires more research and a greater understanding of drug disposition and action within the maternal-fetal placental unit. Thus this area of investigation needs to be expanded. This plea for study occurs at a time when societal and political attitudes are decidedly against human fetal research. We must all work together – obstetricians, pediatricians, prospective mothers and fathers, as well as others who are concerned with the future generations of healthy citizens – to turn this attitude around and resolve this difficult situation.

Index